# ABOUT THE AUTHOR

Meet Lee Holmes, the force behind all things supercharged. She's a qualified clinical nutritionist, yoga and meditation teacher, wholefoods chef and author of the bestselling Supercharged Food series. Her 11 books include *Nature's Way to Healing*, *Heal Your Gut* and the page-turner *Supercharge Your Life*.

When she's not whipping up gut-friendly concoctions in her kitchen, you'll find Lee running her successful online health programs, 'Heal Your Gut' and 'Fast Your Way to Wellness'. She's a regular columnist for *Wellbeing* magazine, and a regular on ABC Radio in Australia. Lee's articles have been published across the globe in prestigious publications like *The Times*, *The Telegraph*, *The Guardian*, *The Daily Express* and *The Australian*.

Lee's website, superchargeyourgut.com, is a gut health haven offering powders and blends including the popular Love Your Gut powder. And her award-winning cooking blog, superchargedfood.com, is a treasure trove of SOLE food: sustainable, organic, local and ethical. You'll find drool-worthy recipes, tantalising information, nutrition news, product reviews and menu-planning ideas that will make your tastebuds tingle.

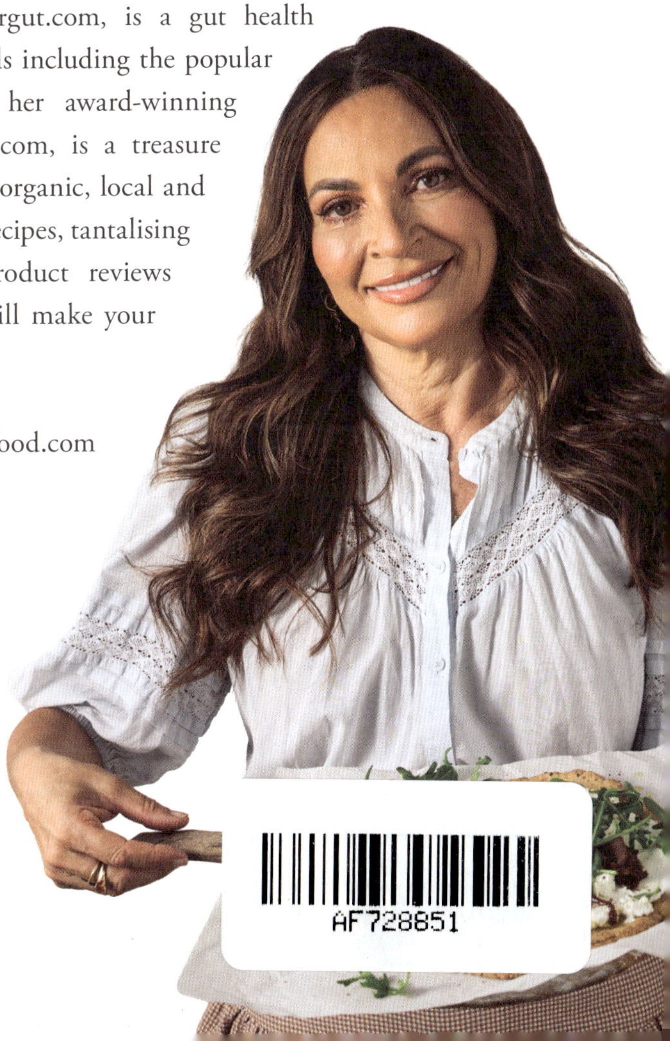

Contact Lee at lee@superchargedfood.com

Follow her adventures at:

- Instagram: leesupercharged
- Facebook: superchargedfood
- YouTube: leesupercharged
- TikTok: superchargedfood

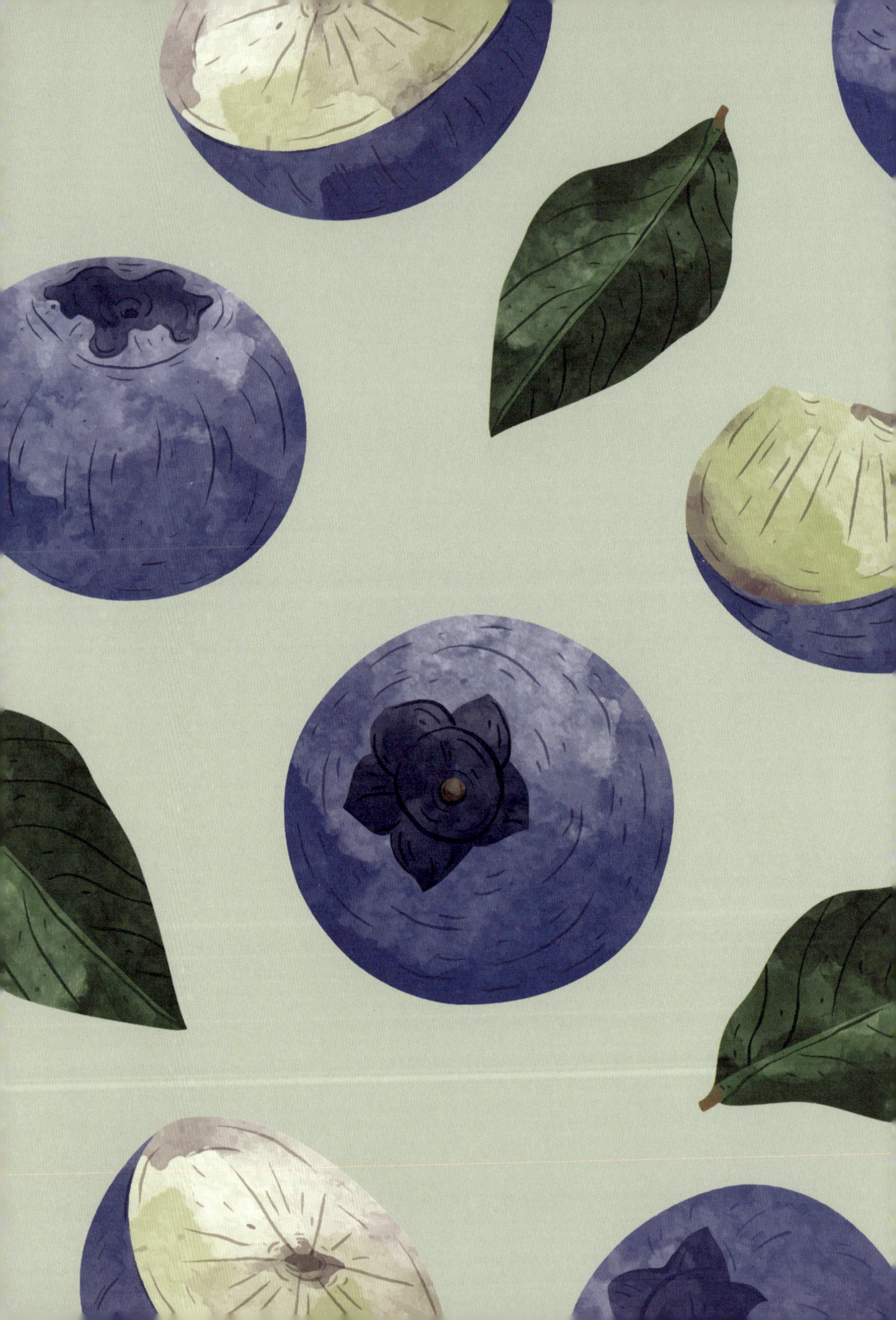

A DELICIOUS guide with 60 RECIPES and the latest BREAKTHROUGHS in inflammation research

# EAT TO HEAL

**Lee Holmes**

ROCKPOOL

DEDICATION

*I dedicate this book and my deepest gratitude to my daughter, Tamsin, who is everything and more.*

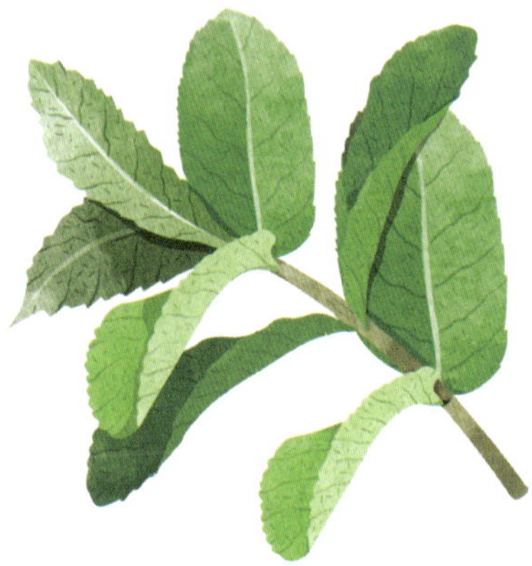

A Rockpool book
PO Box 252
Summer Hill
NSW 2130
Australia

rockpoolpublishing.com
Follow us! rockpoolpublishing
Tag your images with #rockpoolpublishing

ISBN: 9781922468147

Published in 2026 by Rockpool Publishing


Design and typesetting by Sara Lindberg, Rockpool Publishing
Edited by Jessica Cox
Photography by Rob Palmer
Recipes created by Tamsin Holmes @tasteoftamsin
Styling by Vanessa Austin, vanessaaustin.com
Food preparation by Miche Bloch and Emma Norton
Make-up by Louise Antonjuk

Note: The information in this book is for informational purposes only and not intended as a substitute for professional medical advice, diagnosis, or treatment. Always seek the advice of your health practitioner before undertaking a new health care regimen.

NATIONAL LIBRARY OF AUSTRALIA
A catalogue record for this book is available from the National Library of Australia

Printed and bound in China
10 9 8 7 6 5 4 3 2 1

# CONTENTS

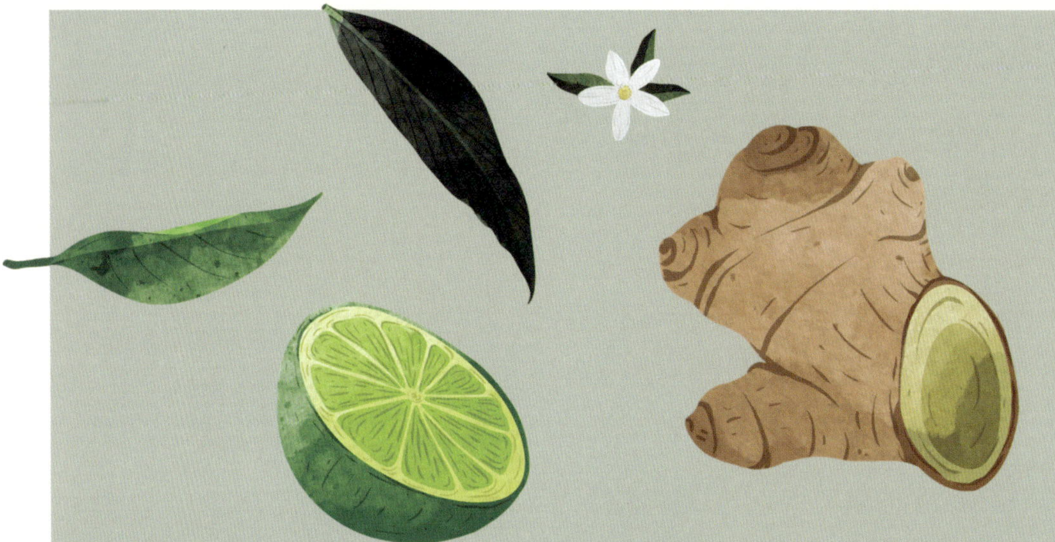

# YOUR KITCHEN IS YOUR MEDICINE CABINET

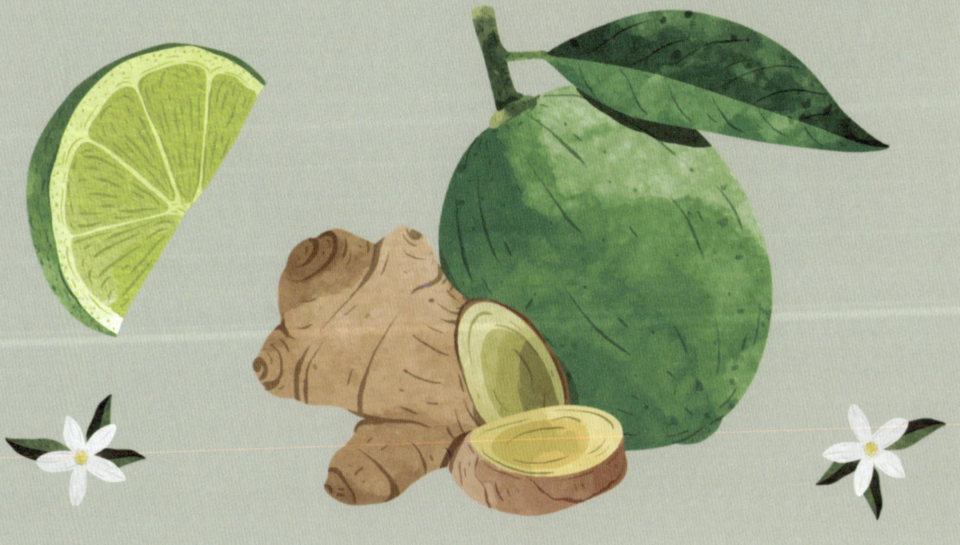

Tired, achy and fed up? This book is for you.

Perhaps this book is in your hands because something doesn't feel quite right. Maybe you've been told 'everything looks normal' on your tests, even though your body is screaming otherwise. Or you've accepted that feeling shattered, achy and foggy-headed is just part of getting older (spoiler alert: it's not).

Imagine waking up feeling truly rested – the kind of rest where you actually want to get out of bed, not just hit snooze for the fifth time. Picture your mind as sharp as a tack, your body energised and free from persistent aches. Instead of dragging yourself through the day like a smartphone on low-battery mode, you feel a sense of ease – your body working with you not staging a daily rebellion.

This isn't some far-fetched fantasy. As a clinical nutritionist, I've witnessed countless patients transform their lives by understanding one critical piece of the wellness puzzle: inflammation. When we reduce inflammation, we open the door to a life that's vibrant, joyful and full of possibility. And yes, that includes being able to open that stubborn jar of sauerkraut without calling for backup.

In this book, I'll help you understand inflammation and its profound impact on your health. Whether you're battling those baffling symptoms that leave doctors puzzled; wrestling with chronic conditions; or feeling trapped in cycles of low mood, anxiety or mental fog when you know you're capable of so much more, you're in the right place. This book is your roadmap to understanding the fascinating connections among inflammation and your gut, mind and body – and more importantly, how to get them all playing nicely together again.

I'll guide you step by step through what's driving your health issues and show you how to shift from feeling depleted, overwhelmed or emotionally flat to feeling genuinely alive and mentally sharp. Food isn't just fuel, it's your most powerful medicine, and your kitchen is the pharmacy you don't need a prescription for. So before you reach for the supplements, swing open those pantry doors! Every delicious bite in this book is like a little doctor's appointment for your insides, carefully hand-picked to repair, refresh and

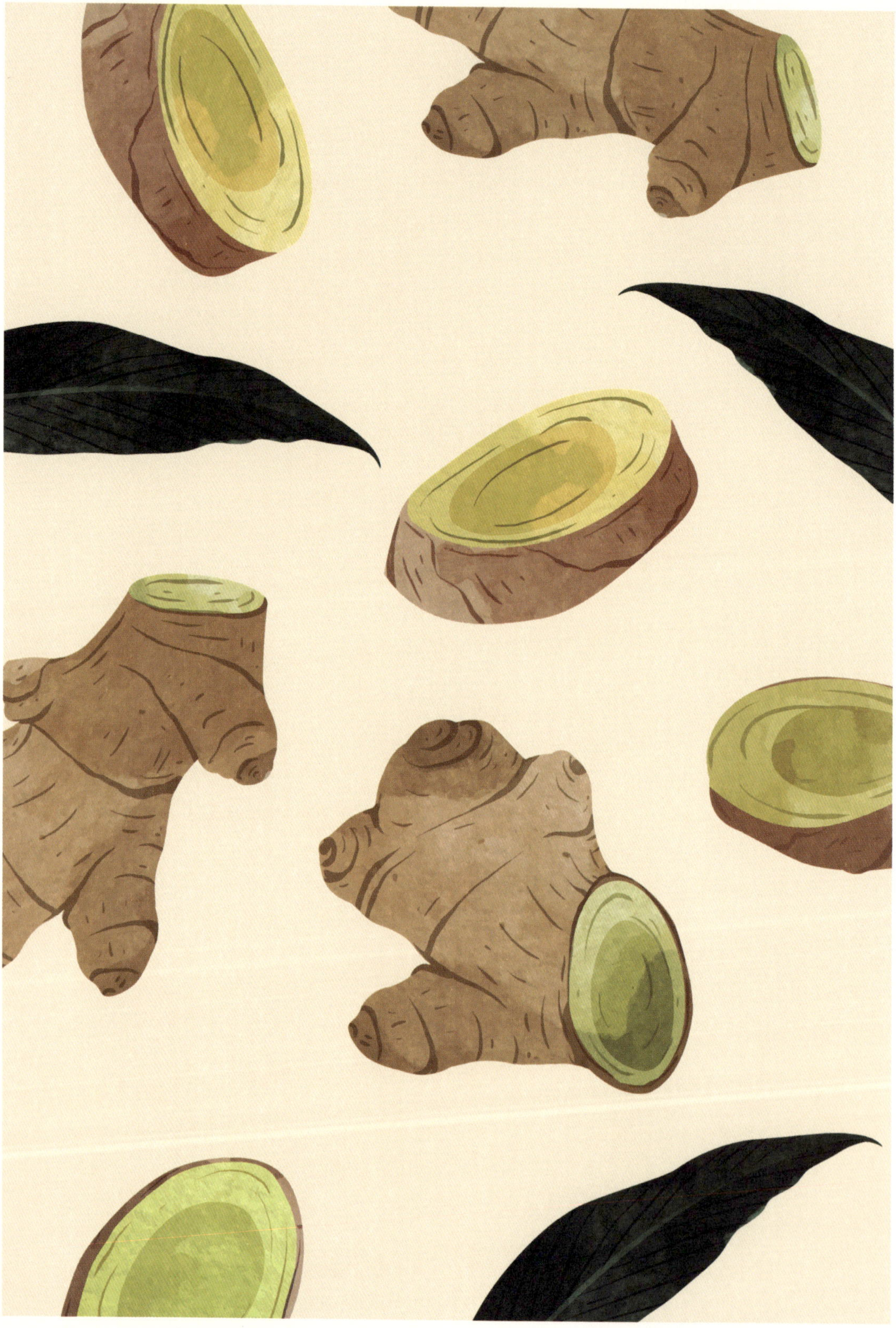

heal your body from the gut upwards, and the inside out, one tasty spoonful at a time.

Together, we'll uncover the root causes of your symptoms and create a clear path towards the vibrant health you deserve, using the transformative power of anti-inflammatory nutrition. The mouth-watering recipes ahead are your daily prescription for cellular renewal and nervous system restoration.

No more accepting 'tired and fed up' as your normal – it's time to heal, rewrite your health story and live free from inflammation. Prepare to calm your nervous system and energise every single cell, one delicious and healing meal at a time!

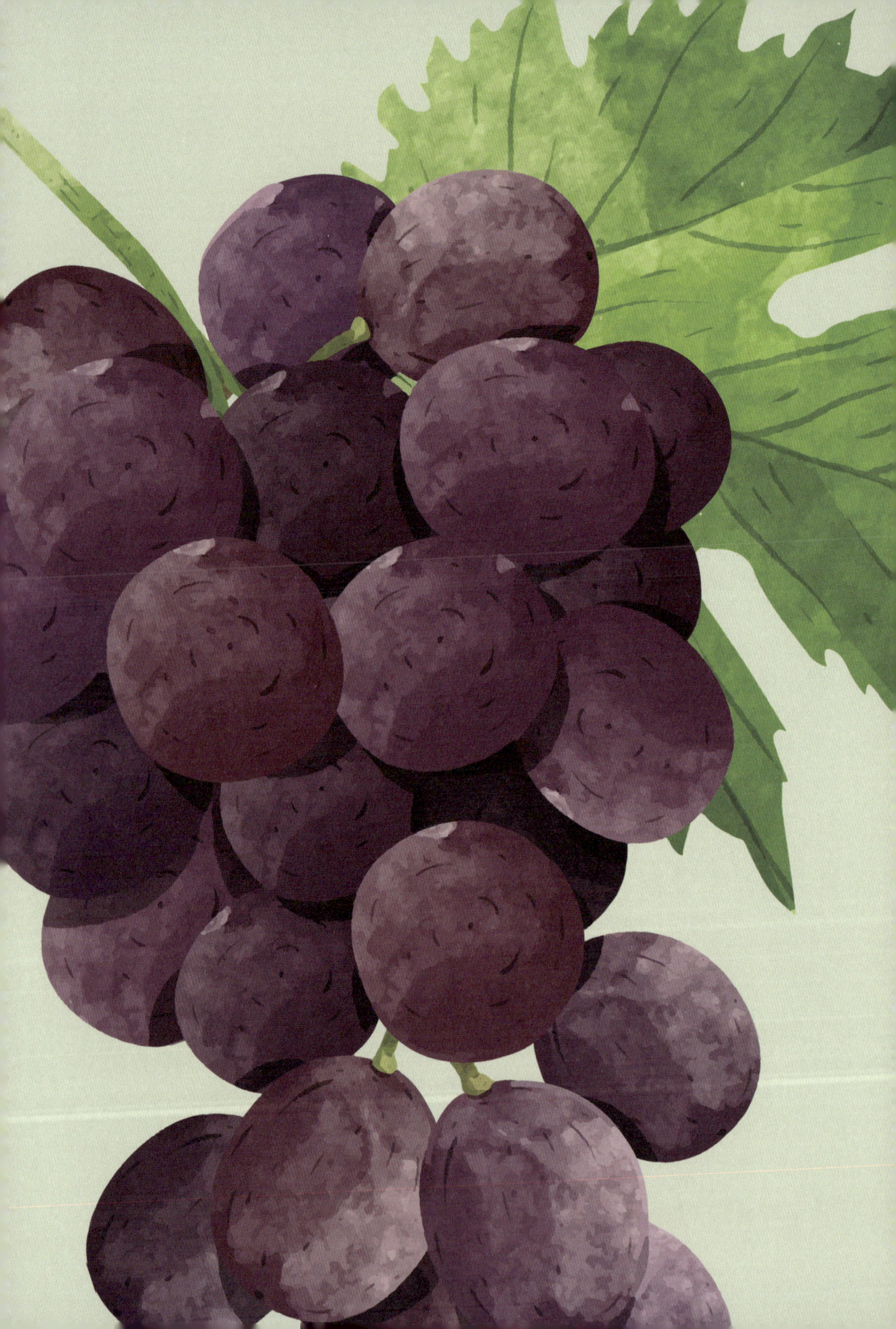

PART 1

# INFLAMMATION, THE BODY'S DOUBLE-EDGED SWORD

Understanding inflammation is the foundation of your healing journey. You'll discover how inflammation can both protect and harm your body, setting the stage for everything that follows. By identifying what inflammation is, when it becomes chronic and what drives it, you're taking the first step towards reducing inflammation in your body. This knowledge will empower you to make informed decisions that support cellular health and prepare your nervous system for the healing strategies in this book. Before we can tame inflammation, however, we need to understand this fascinating biological process – your body's most brilliant double-edged sword.

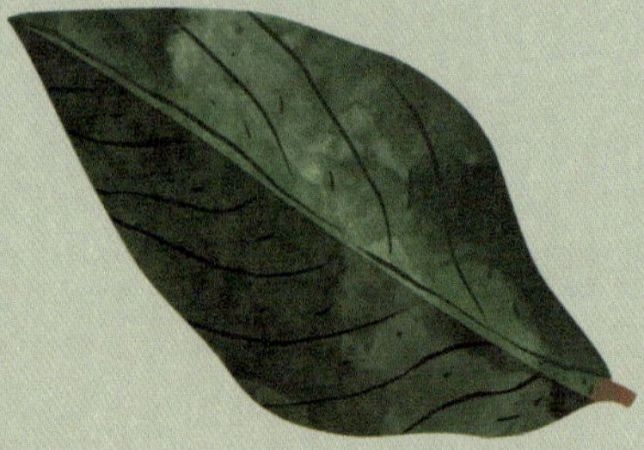

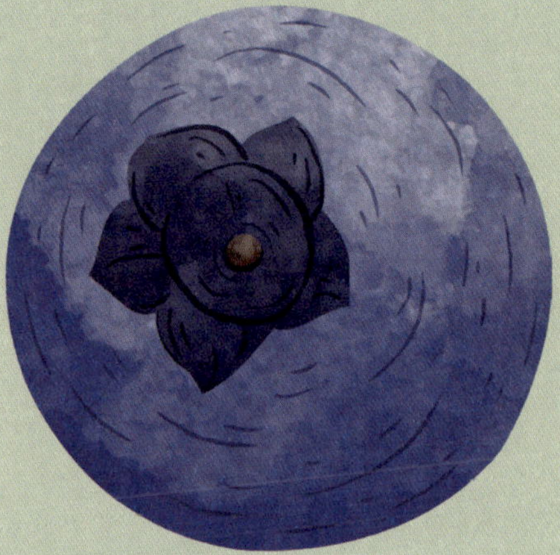

CHAPTER 1

# WHAT IS INFLAMMATION?

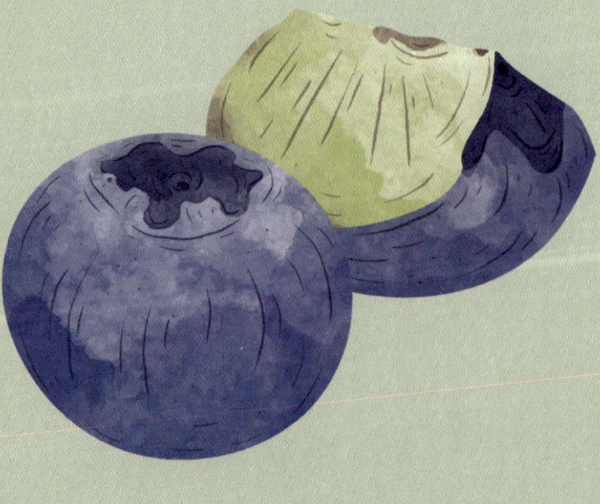

Inflammation is one of the most talked-about topics in health and wellness, yet it often feels like an intimidating concept. Here's the thing: inflammation isn't always the villain it's made out to be. It's your body's built-in superhero, rushing to protect and heal when you scrape your knee, catch a cold or twist your ankle.

When you injure yourself, the redness, heat and swelling that follow are all signs that your body is working to repair the damage. This is acute inflammation – a short-term response that's essential for survival. Without it, cuts wouldn't heal, infections could spread unchecked and our bodies would be defenceless.

But what happens when inflammation hangs around too long and overstays its welcome? That's where things get tricky. Chronic inflammation is like an overzealous security guard who starts seeing threats everywhere, even when there aren't any. It's subtle, often silent and can simmer for years – a slow burn that can quietly undermine your health.

## YOUR BODY'S EMERGENCY RESPONSE CENTRE

Imagine your body as a bustling city with an emergency response centre where millions of tiny specialists work round the clock to keep you healthy. When a threat emerges – a microscopic pathogen, physical injury or environmental toxin – this sophisticated system springs into action with precision.

**Cytokines** are like text messages zipping between immune cells, either ramping up the emergency response or calling for calm. Some cytokines such as tumour necrosis factor (TNF) and interleukin-6 act as emergency alerts, while others (like interleukin-10) play the peacemaker, preventing your immune system from going overboard.

**Interleukins** are your immune system's air traffic controllers. If cytokines are the messages, interleukins are the dispatchers, coordinating your white blood cells and managing both the intensity and duration of inflammation. When they malfunction – as in conditions like lupus – these dispatchers start sending out too many distress signals, leading to inflammatory chaos.

**C-reactive protein** (CRP) is your body's fire alarm system. When inflammation strikes, elevated CRP levels act like a red flag, warning of chronic inflammation and potentially increasing your risk of heart disease and autoimmune conditions.

## ACUTE INFLAMMATION: Your body's rescue mission

You can think of acute inflammation as a life-saving process, a precisely choreographed rescue mission unfolding in your body. When you suffer a cut or encounter an infection, the following sequence unfolds:

- White blood cells rush to the site as first responders.
- Increased blood flow causes warmth and redness (vasodilation) at the affected area.
- Swelling helps deliver immune factors and nutrients needed for tissue repair and defence.
- Pain signals encourage you to protect the area.
- Healing begins, ensuring your full recovery.

It's a testament to your body's innate intelligence – rapidly detecting threats and orchestrating an effective response.

When the threat is neutralised and healing is complete, your body performs one final masterstroke: the inflammatory response switches off, returning tissues to their normal state. This elegant resolution ensures that inflammation doesn't overstay its welcome, allowing your body to return to optimal function without any lingering effects.

Inflammation is also closely linked to your fight-or-flight response. Stress hormones like cortisol and adrenaline can amplify or suppress immune activity, influencing how your body reacts to perceived dangers. The same protective mechanism can become profoundly destructive, however, when it loses its regulatory balance.

## THE MOLECULAR CONVERSATION

Inflammation is a complex molecular conversation happening inside your body. When it functions properly, those cytokines, interleukins and inflammatory markers work in perfect harmony. But when the conversation becomes distorted – when the messages get stuck on repeat or the signals become scrambled – your body loses its ability to distinguish between genuine threats and everyday encounters.

I experience this firsthand during mast cell activation syndrome flare-ups. During these episodes, I can almost feel my body's molecular conversation spiralling out of control, suddenly reacting to triggers (certain foods, environmental factors or even stress) I'm usually fine with. This personal health crisis became my greatest teacher. It drove me to dive deep into nutritional science and ultimately qualify as a clinical nutritionist. What began as a desperate search for answers about my own health puzzle transformed into a passion for helping others decode their body's messages and find their path to healing through targeted nutrition.

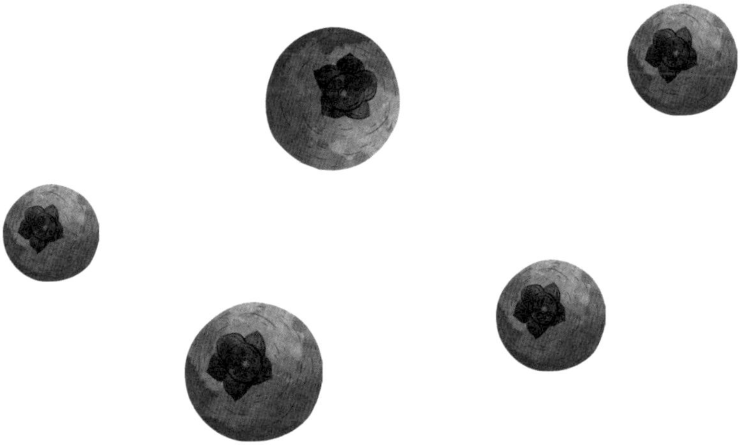

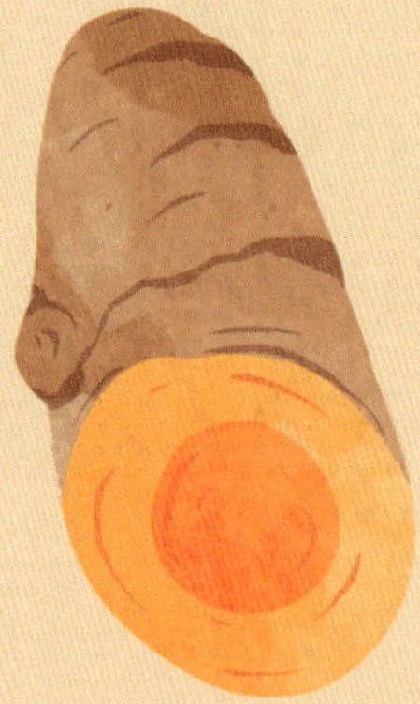

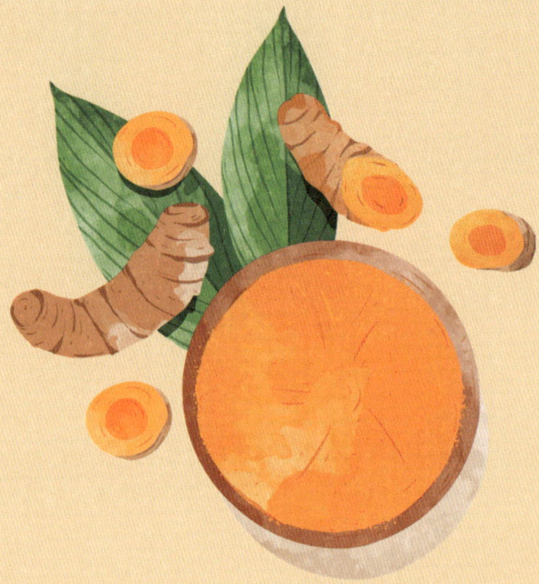

CHAPTER 2

# WHEN INFLAMMATION BECOMES CHRONIC

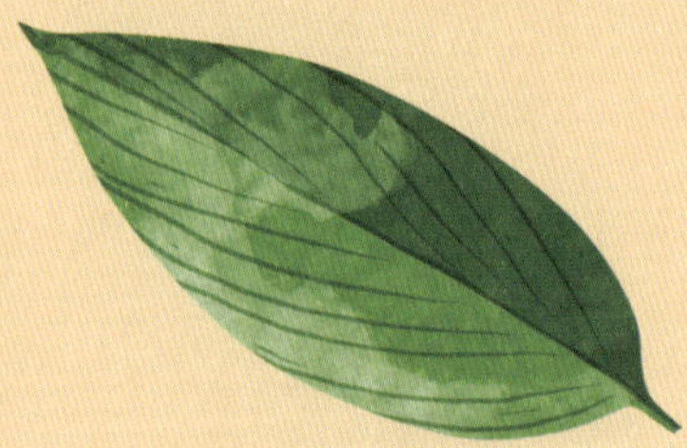

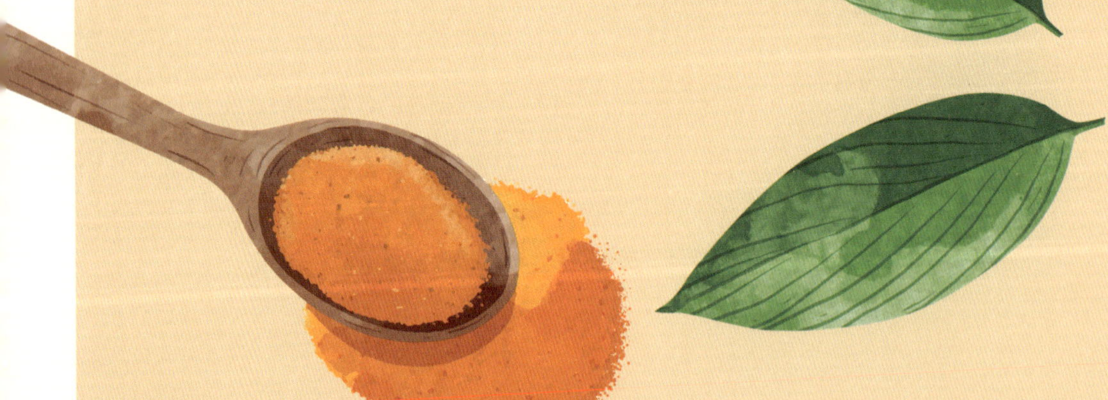

## WHEN YOUR PROTECTIVE SYSTEM GOES HAYWIRE

While acute inflammation is your body's life-saving mechanism, chronic inflammation is a critical breakdown of this natural protective system. Your immune system's security guard has forgotten to clock off – instead of a precise, targeted response, your body's stuck on perpetual high alert.

This sustained inflammatory state emerges from a complex interplay of genetic, environmental and lifestyle factors. Modern life with its processed foods, chronic stress, environmental toxins and sedentary habits creates the perfect conditions for inflammatory chaos. It's like living in a house where the smoke detector never stops beeping, even when there's no fire.

## WHO'S IN THE INFLAMMATION HOT SEAT?

Let's see who might need to pay extra attention to their inflammatory levels. Unfortunately, some of us are more prone to inflammation, while others have made lifestyle choices that are about as helpful as a paper umbrella in a storm.

If you have pre-existing conditions like diabetes, autoimmune disorders and metabolic syndrome, you already have inflammation simmering away in the background like a forgotten pot of porridge on the stovetop. Then there's the joy of ageing. Along with grey hair and creaky knees, our bodies also are adept at ramping up inflammation over time, making our blood vessels inflexible.

Genetics can throw a massive spanner in the works too; some bodies handle cholesterol and inflammation less efficiently. And lifestyle choices – smoking, eating ultra-processed foods, drinking excessive alcohol and having chronic stress levels – are like throwing petrol on your inflammatory fire.

## INFLAMMATION UNDER THE RADAR

Chronic inflammation is sneaky because it can fly under the radar. This silent progression occurs through microscopic changes that accumulate imperceptibly – CRP increases incrementally rather than dramatically, and cellular damage happens at scales too small for immediate detection but significant for long-term health.

You might notice subtle, seemingly unrelated symptoms creeping in: persistent fatigue that no amount of coffee can fix, brain fog that makes you forget why you walked into a room (again) and mysterious weight fluctuations despite your best efforts. These aren't random health hiccups, they're interconnected signals of systemic inflammatory disruption.

It's like your body's group chat has gone haywire. Instead of resolving issues, every system keeps asking, 'Are you still experiencing this problem?' Meanwhile, your metabolism has gone quiet, your brain is constantly buffering and your energy levels are as reliable as Wi-Fi in an underground carpark.

## SPOTTING THE RED FLAGS

Your body often sends warning signals long before major issues arise. Here are some sneaky signs inflammation might be taking hold:

- Persistent fatigue that sleep doesn't fix
- Unexplained weight changes despite consistent habits
- Digestive irregularities that seem to come from nowhere
- Mood fluctuations that feel out of character
- Recurring infections that suggest compromised immunity
- Slow wound healing

If several of these symptoms sound familiar, consider it your body's polite way of requesting attention, a signal that underlying inflammatory activity needs addressing.

### Testing for inflammation

If those warning signs are ringing bells, getting some objective data can help confirm what your body's already telling you. Two key blood tests can reveal inflammation lurking beneath the surface:

**CRP (C-reactive protein)** is your body's warning system. Produced by the liver, CRP levels rise in response to systemic inflammation, even when no obvious symptoms are present. It highlights underlying inflammatory activity that might otherwise go unnoticed. Checking your CRP levels is one way to assess whether your body is in an inflammatory state.

**ESR (erythrocyte sedimentation rate)** is often tested alongside CRP. This blood test measures how quickly red blood cells settle at the bottom of a test tube, providing an indirect indication of inflammation levels. Higher ESR results suggest increased inflammation, because inflammatory conditions cause red blood cells to clump together and settle more rapidly.

Understanding inflammation is the first step in taking control of your health. Once you grasp how this complex system works – both for and against you – you can begin to work *with* your body's natural processes rather than against them.

## THE INFLAMMATORY BALANCING ACT

The key to vibrant health lies in maintaining the delicate balance between pro-inflammatory and anti-inflammatory responses in your body. When this balance tips towards persistent inflammation, it can contribute to a cascade of modern health challenges: cardiovascular problems, diabetes, autoimmune conditions and mental health struggles. The good news? Understanding this process is the first step to take back control.

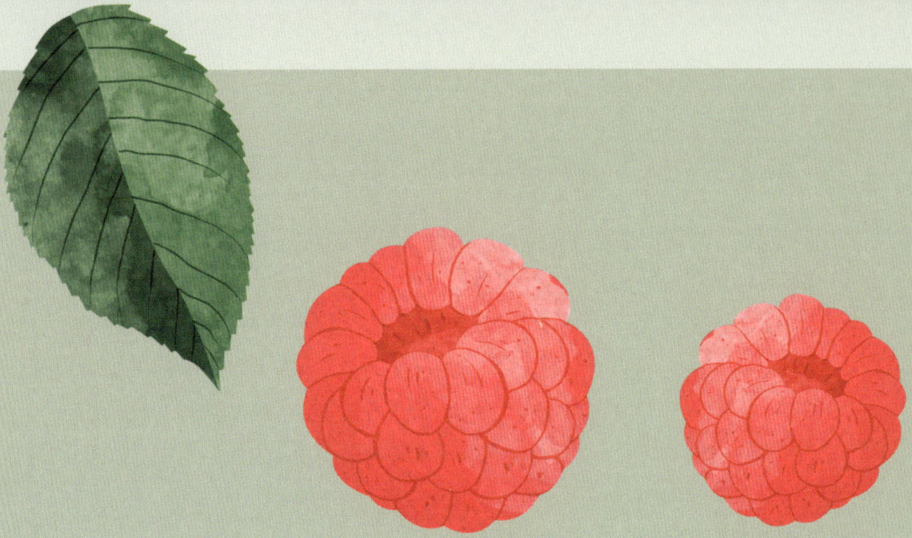

CHAPTER 3

# WHAT CAUSES CHRONIC INFLAMMATION?

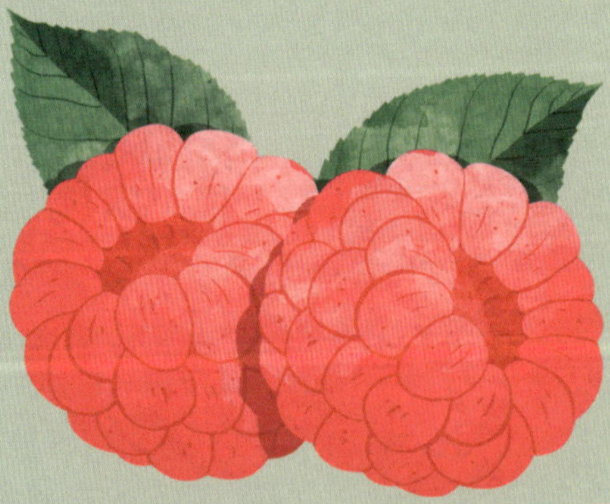

Chronic inflammation doesn't emerge randomly but is triggered by a complex interplay of factors that shape the body's immune response over time. While genetics may predispose some individuals to higher inflammatory tendencies, factors like environmental exposures, nutrient-deficient modern diets, sedentary lifestyle habits and psychological stressors are often the real ignition sources – turning low-grade inflammation into a persistent, health-disrupting force.

In this chapter, I'll break down the key triggers that keep inflammation simmering beneath the surface, how they interact and what you can do to minimise their impact on your long-term health.

## HOW GENETICS AND MODERN LIFE FUEL INFLAMMATION

Your system can't function at its best when inflammation is running rampant. It's like a city-wide protest where every cell is holding up tiny 'Down with oxidative stress!' placards. Here are the usual suspects that can keep your inflammatory fires burning:

- Genetics
- Mental health issues
- Gut health issues
- Diet and lifestyle
- Environment

# ❶ THE GENETICS OF INFLAMMATION: Your cellular blueprint

Our genetic landscape is as unique as our fingerprints, determining how our immune system responds to life's challenges. Some people inherit genetic variations that make them more prone to inflammatory responses, like having a sensitive smoke alarm that goes off when you burn toast.

Your genes aren't your destiny; they're more like a piano, and you decide which keys to play with your lifestyle choices. Traumatic experiences can also reprogram immune cells, making them overreact or underreact to future threats, creating chronic inflammation where your body remains on high alert even when no real danger exists.

## Zombie cells: The creepy houseguests of ageing

Over time some cells stop performing their tasks but still linger like unwelcome guests, causing dysfunction. These senescent cells are nicknamed 'zombie cells'.

Zombie cells release inflammatory signals that disrupt neighbouring cells and fuel chronic diseases. Like an old factory continuously leaking toxic fumes, senescent cells stoke the fires of inflammation, weakening tissues and increasing your susceptibility to disease.

## The cellular energy crisis

Chronic inflammation disrupts your mitochondria – the tiny energy factories within each cell. It causes adenosine triphosphate (ATP) production to decline, leaving you feeling fatigued and slowing your body's repair processes. It's like having your power stations running at half capacity while your city's energy demands remain the same.

Chronic inflammation also accelerates telomere shortening. These protective caps on chromosome ends naturally wear down over time, but inflammation speeds up this process, impairing cellular function and causing premature ageing.

The key lies in working with your genetic blueprint rather than against it, creating an environment where your cells can thrive rather than merely survive.

# ❷ MENTAL HEALTH AND YOUR BODY'S INVISIBLE FIRE STARTERS

When chronic stress, anxiety, depression or trauma come knocking, your body floods with cortisol. Over time, this hormonal chaos fans the flames of inflammation faster than gossip spreads through a village.

## When your stress system gets stuck in overdrive

During prolonged psychological stress, your hypothalamic–pituitary–adrenal axis is chronically activated. This axis is a major neuroendocrine system that regulates your stress response, mood, digestion, immune function, energy metabolism and other vital processes. Cortisol, traditionally an anti-inflammatory hormone, becomes dysregulated. Under normal circumstances cortisol acts like a skilled negotiator, calming inflammatory responses. But prolonged stress creates a biochemical environment where cortisol loses its effectiveness, and starts promoting rather than suppressing inflammation.

It's like having a fire chief who's been working non-stop for months – they eventually start making poor decisions and accidentally pour petrol on the flames instead of water.

## The mind–body highway

Mental health struggles trigger a cascade of events:

- Your sympathetic nervous system fires up.
- Cortisol floods your system.
- Inflammatory molecules like interleukin-6, TNF and CRP (your body's short-term response to injury) help to contain and repair damage.

If the production of these short-term inflammatory molecules becomes uncontrolled or prolonged, they create systemic inflammation, disrupting normal blood flow and tissue function and increasing the risk of chronic disease. These long-term patterns can persist long after the initial stressor has passed.

## Your body's inconvenient memory bank

Unresolved trauma, particularly adverse childhood experiences, has been linked to long-term alterations in immune function. You become more susceptible to chronic inflammatory diseases, including autoimmune disorders, cardiovascular conditions and metabolic syndrome (for more, see Chapter 6).

# ❸ GUT HEALTH: When your internal security goes AWOL

Your gut is ground zero for inflammation. The lining of your gut is naturally semi-permeable, letting nutrients from food pass through into your bloodstream so they can nourish your cells. At the same time, it acts as a barrier to keep out pathogens, toxins and waste materials. When this delicate lining becomes damaged (a condition known as 'leaky gut') unwanted particles can slip through, triggering inflammation and a wide range of health issues (for more, see Chapter 5).

## The gut–brain conversation

When stress activates your hypothalamic–pituitary–adrenal axis, it disrupts the peaceful community of microbes living in your gut. This disruption leads to increased intestinal permeability (leaky gut), allowing troublemakers like toxic bacteria to sneak into your bloodstream and add fuel to the inflammatory fire.

This two-way street between your gut and brain, facilitated by the vagus nerve and various signalling pathways, is a constant conversation between your mind and body (for more, see Chapter 5).

## ④ DIET AND LIFESTYLE: Your inflammation superpower or supervillain?

Your food choices can either feed the flames or act as a fire extinguisher. That late-night takeaway might taste heavenly, but those refined carbohydrates, trans fats and processed foods are adding to your inflammatory bonfire. The good news? It can be reversed when you eat to heal.

### INFLAMMATION-FIGHTING FOODS: YOUR CELLULAR FIRE DEPARTMENT

Every bite matters. Fill your plate with colourful vegetables, wild-caught fish and spices like turmeric. Foods rich in antioxidants, healthy fats and phytonutrients extinguish chronic inflammation and protect your cells from damage.

### The modern food chaos

In my clinic, I've witnessed remarkable transformations in clients struggling with persistent brain fog, afternoon energy crashes and joint pain once they learned how to lower their inflammation levels. Research shows processed foods can increase inflammatory markers like CRP by up to 40%, while antioxidant-rich whole foods help to maintain the body's delicate balance and supercharge cellular function.

The modern diet of processed foods, refined sugars and artificial additives is a radical departure from the nutritional environments that shaped human biology. Processed foods aren't just empty calories – they come with a side order of chaos. Refined sugars spike blood glucose levels, sending your metabolic system on a roller-coaster ride and generating advanced glycation end products (AGEs). AGEs are aptly named because they accelerate ageing and inflammation.

## When movement is optional

Sedentary lifestyles compound these dietary challenges. Our sit-more, move-less culture makes our metabolism sluggish. Metabolic stagnation prevents the muscles from producing anti-inflammatory myokines – protective compounds that normally help keep inflammation in check.

Just like an unused treadmill gathers dust in the corner, an idle body becomes a playground for chronic inflammation. When we don't move, we aren't supercharging our cells with the anti-inflammatory benefits of physical activity.

## The nutrient depletion crisis

Throughout my years in practice, I've found that nutritional deficiencies further fuel inflammatory processes. Modern farming practices have diminished the nutrient density of foods, creating widespread micronutrient deficiencies that compromise the immune system.

Critical minerals like zinc, selenium and magnesium all modulate inflammatory responses and keep the nervous system calm. When these become depleted, it's like trying to conduct an orchestra when half the instruments are missing – the whole performance suffers.

## Your path to anti-inflammatory living

Every meal presents an opportunity to either fan the flames of inflammation or douse them – to eat to heal rather than harm. In Part 3, I'll share my personalised Mediterranean, anti-inflammatory plan (MAP) approach, exploring how a targeted diet with nutrient-rich foods can help restore these critical micronutrients, calm your nervous system and supercharge every cell in your body.

Your fork is one of the most powerful healing tools for transforming your health – let's learn how to wield it like the inflammation-fighting ninja it can be.

# ⑤ ENVIRONMENT

The invisible troublemakers in our modern world are teeming with inflammatory provocateurs that our ancient ancestors never encountered. From air pollution outside to the cleaning products under your sink, modern life is a chemical cocktail.

Industrial chemicals, heavy metals and synthetic compounds interact with our cellular machinery like gatecrashers at a party, disrupting the body's systems. Your body is trying to filter all this out, but it's like asking a tea strainer to catch bowling balls. Given our modern exposure to toxins and microplastics, future archaeologists might classify us as a new species – *Homo plasticus*!

Our environment should help to regulate inflammation, yet it now contains an overwhelming array of toxins that increase our body's inflammatory burden. The Industrial Revolution brought rapid advancements but also introduced new chemicals and pollutants. After World War II, economic growth accelerated this trend, embedding synthetic materials, pesticides and additives into everyday life. Scientists only began uncovering their long-term health consequences decades later but by then, these toxins were unavoidable.

Picture your body as an ecosystem, each cell a worker bee operating in finely tuned harmony. Now imagine a swarm of gnats disrupting that ecosystem, irritating the workers and causing chaos. That's what environmental toxins do.

Even seemingly harmless items harbour hidden toxins. That disposable paper coffee cup has a plastic lining made with bisphenol A (BPA) or substitutes, which leach into hot beverages. They may also contain per- and polyfluoroalkyl substances (PFAS) for water resistance. Even reusable plastic or metal cups can introduce harmful compounds to the body. Over time, these exposures overwhelm the body's detoxification systems, leading to chronic inflammation.

## The invisible pollutants that fuel inflammation

Environmental toxins trigger immune overactivity, increase cytokine production, promote oxidative stress, disrupt gut microbiota and interfere with hormone balance. These biochemical effects contribute to conditions like autoimmune diseases, metabolic disorders, brain fog, infertility and chronic fatigue.

Common culprits:

- **Tap water** may contain chlorine, fluoride, PFAS (which can bioaccumulate) and heavy metals such as lead or mercury from ageing pipes or environmental pollution.
- **Beauty products** may have phthalates, parabens or formaldehyde releasers, even 'natural' ones. These can act as endocrine disruptors or allergens.
- **Takeaway food containers** can leach harmful substances such as BPA, phthalates, plasticisers and microplastics into food, especially when heated.
- **Green smoothies** – I kid you not! Pesticides on produce like spinach and kale can harm gut bacteria.
- **Plastic blender cups** can leach microplastics and chemicals like BPA, which are linked to hormonal disruption, especially with repeated use and heat.
- **Almond milk** may contain carrageenan, linked to gut inflammation.

## Where toxins hide and how they affect you

**Modern homes often trap airborne pollutants.** Mould spores release mycotoxins that disrupt immune function. Volatile organic compounds (VOCs) from furniture, paints and cleaning products irritate respiratory pathways and interfere with endocrine balance.

**Industrial emissions, vehicle exhaust, home wood-burning stoves and pesticides** contribute to air pollution. Fine particulate matter (PM2.5) has been linked to increased inflammatory markers like CRP and interleukin-6, raising risks for cardiovascular disease and neuroinflammation.

**Heavy metals (lead, mercury, arsenic)** can contaminate tap water and foods, disrupting cellular function and increasing oxidative stress. Consuming pesticides on non-organic produce harm gut microbiota, while microplastics found in bottled water and seafood induce immune responses.

**Everyday items like cosmetics, cleaning supplies and furniture** often contain endocrine-disrupting chemicals, which interfere with hormone function and contribute to systemic inflammation.

## SIMPLE STEPS TO DETOXIFY YOUR LIFE

**To minimise your exposure, you need to purify, eliminate and consume mindfully. Here's how:**

| | |
|---|---|
| **1. Improve indoor air quality.** | Use HEPA (high efficiency particulate arresting) filters: H13 or higher, and open windows regularly. |
| | Add air-purifying houseplants like peace lilies, spider plants and snake plants. |
| **2. Choose safer cleaning products.** | Opt for products made with vinegar, baking soda and essential oils instead of harsh chemicals. |
| **3. Filter your water.** | Invest in a high-quality filtration system to remove contaminants. Have filtered showers. |
| **4. Prioritise organic and whole foods.** | Choose organic, particularly for the 'Dirty Dozen' list of pesticide-heavy produce. |
| | Avoid processed foods with artificial additives. |
| **5. Use non-toxic personal care products.** | Choose fragrance-free products verified by the EWG (Environmental Working Group). |
| | Avoid items with parabens, sulfates and synthetic fragrances. |
| **6. Reduce plastic exposure.** | Use glass, stainless steel or silicone containers instead of plastic. |
| | Avoid microwaving food in plastic containers. |

## DETOX POWER: How to support your body's built-in clean-up crew

Reducing your exposure is just one part of the equation. Supporting detoxification pathways enhances your body's ability to eliminate toxins efficiently.

1. **The liver detoxes the system in two phases:**
    - Phase I converts toxins into intermediate compounds.
    - Phase II neutralises these compounds and excretes them.

#### HOW TO SUPPORT:

Eat sulfur-rich foods (garlic, onions, cruciferous vegetables).
Supplement with glutathione and milk thistle.

2. **A diverse gut microbiome breaks down toxins and prevents reabsorption.**
    - Eat fibre-rich foods, fermented foods and prebiotics.
    - Stay hydrated to support elimination.
3. **The lymphatic system clears waste and toxins.**
    - Practise dry brushing and rebounding.
    - Use infrared saunas for enhanced detoxification.

Think of supporting your detox pathways like giving your body a gentle nudge (not a slap) because even your liver prefers a spa day over a boxing match.

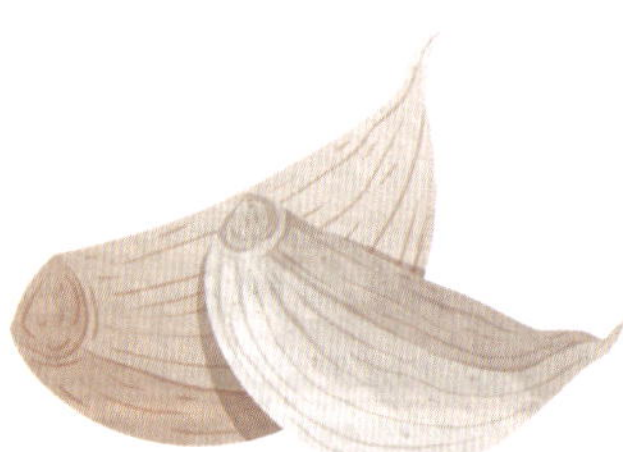

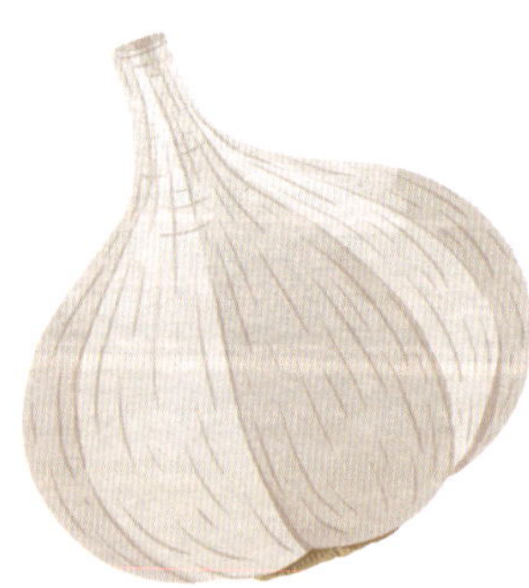

## CLEAN LIVING: Building a low-toxin lifestyle that sticks

Reducing your toxin exposure is about making small, intentional changes for long-term health. Here are steps you can take:

- Replace conventional products with non-toxic alternatives over time.
- Educate yourself on common toxins and their sources.
- Prioritise clean, locally sourced foods.
- Create a toxin-free sleep environment with organic bedding.
- Regularly clean your home to prevent mould and dust build-up.
- Invest in quality air and water filtration.
- Manage stress because chronic stress impairs detoxification.

While we can't eliminate all toxins, we can dramatically reduce our exposure and strengthen resilience. Small, mindful changes can profoundly impact our inflammation and overall well-being.

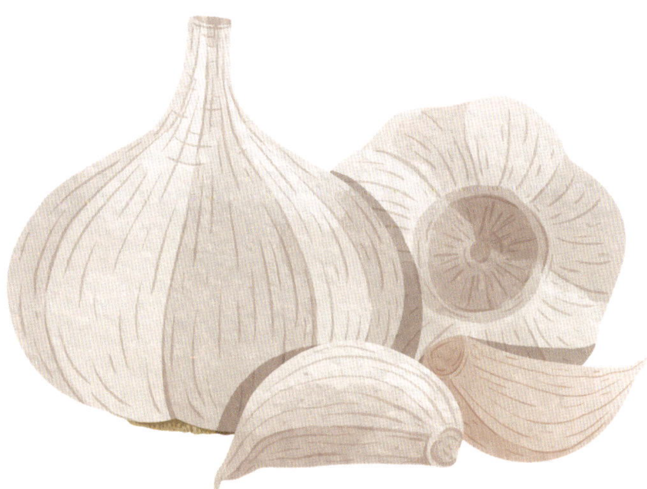

CHAPTER 4

# HOW CHRONIC INFLAMMATION DISRUPTS FROM HEAD TO TOE

Picture your body as a bustling metropolis. Your cardiovascular system is its intricate transport network and your brain is the central command centre, processing information and directing essential functions. Like any thriving city, your body requires smooth-running roads (blood vessels), an efficient healthcare system (immune system) and well-coordinated emergency services (inflammatory responses). But what happens when your city's emergency services stay on high alert for too long? Chronic inflammation turns a normally protective response into a city-wide crisis – clogging arteries, disrupting metabolic pathways and interfering with brain function.

Understanding how inflammation impacts the body and mind is key to creating a healthier, more resilient system – one where your city runs smoothly, your immune defences stay balanced, and your brain remains sharp and protected.

The good news? Research has revealed clear connections between your city's management choices (lifestyle) and its emergency response patterns (inflammation), meaning you have more control than you might think over your body's inflammatory state. By understanding these mechanisms, you can protect not just your heart and metabolism, but also your brain's clarity, resilience and longevity.

## THE CITY'S TRANSPORT CRISIS: Inflammation and cardiovascular disease

Your city's transport network is a vast system of motorways, roads and side streets that ensure essential supplies (oxygen and nutrients) travel smoothly throughout your body. Chronic inflammation is like having endless roadworks, diversions and traffic jams disrupting this vital flow. Formerly smooth, flexible roads become narrowed and rigid, leading to serious circulation problems.

At the heart of this dysfunction is atherosclerosis – troublesome potholes where fatty deposits accumulate along your arterial motorways, restricting traffic flow and increasing the risk of major incidents (heart attacks and strokes). This process begins when the road surface (endothelium) gets damaged by high blood pressure, smoking, toxins and elevated cholesterol levels. Your body's emergency response team (immune cells) rushes to repair the damage, but they often make the problem worse, contributing to ongoing roadworks (plaque accumulation) and traffic disruptions (inflammation).

## Let's have a heart to heart

Research has established strong links between inflammation and cardiovascular disease. Reducing inflammation may be just as important as lowering cholesterol for preventing heart disease. Previously the emphasis was on cholesterol, but scientists are now looking at inflammation as the hidden culprit behind many heart issues.

While high levels of low-density lipoprotein (LDL) cholesterol is a factor, what's happening in the arteries is also important. Chronic inflammation damages blood vessel walls, making them more susceptible to plaque build-up. Studies show that people with high levels of inflammatory markers like CRP are at greater risk of heart attacks even if their cholesterol levels are normal.

## Inflammation's key role in cardiovascular health

Atherosclerosis was once thought to be the result of passive cholesterol accumulation in the arterial walls. More than a century ago, however, Rudolf Virchow observed inflammatory white blood cells within atherosclerotic plaques, hinting at a deeper immunological role. Research has since confirmed that inflammation is a central driver of atherosclerosis.

From the earliest stages of endothelial dysfunction to foam cell formation, plaque growth and ultimately plaque rupture, inflammation orchestrates every step of the disease process.

'The inflammatory process is orchestrating everything from the very beginning of atherosclerosis up to its progression and complications.' Dr Peter Libby, Cardiovascular medicine specialist at Harvard Medical School, says.

Dr Libby emphasises the fundamental role of inflammation in cardiovascular disease from the initial stages of plaque formation to severe complications like heart attacks and strokes.

Recent studies have revealed even more connections. Higher CRP levels are consistently associated with an increased risk of heart attacks, strokes and other cardiovascular complications. CRP is now a standardised biomarker in clinical practice.

Perhaps most intriguingly, emerging research has identified a significant link between gut health and cardiovascular disease through the gut microbiota-derived metabolite trimethylamine N-oxide (TMAO). Elevated TMAO levels are associated with an increased risk of atherosclerotic cardiovascular disease and related complications, including death. These findings suggest that imbalances in gut bacteria can contribute to systemic inflammation and cause plaque to form in the arteries, opening new avenues for treatment and prevention.

The 2017 CANTOS trial proved that reducing inflammation significantly lowers the risk of recurrent cardiovascular events. Patients who received canakinumab (a monoclonal antibody targeting interleukin-1 beta) experienced fewer heart attacks and strokes, even without changes in cholesterol levels. This breakthrough confirmed that chronic inflammation is not just a consequence but a driving force behind heart disease.

Why does this matter for you? It means that managing inflammation through diet, stress reduction and gut health optimisation can be just as – if not more – effective than focusing solely on cholesterol levels.

But the impact of inflammation doesn't stop at the heart; it extends to the brain. Just as inflammation clogs arteries, it also infiltrates neural pathways, leading to neuroinflammation. The same inflammatory markers (CRP and interleukin-6) linked to heart disease are also implicated in cognitive decline, depression and neurodegenerative disorders like Alzheimer's and Parkinson's diseases.

In other words: if your arteries are inflamed, your brain likely is too. Understanding this heart–brain connection is key to preventing cognitive decline, mood imbalances and long-term neurological disease.

## BRAIN ON FIRE: Neuroinflammation's role in mental health

The brain is often considered a well-protected control centre, shielded by the blood–brain barrier and supported by an intricate network of neurons and neurotransmitters. But chronic inflammation can breach these defences, silently reshaping brain function and increasing the risk of cognitive decline, mood disorders and neurodegeneration.

It's not just background noise; chronic inflammation actively interferes with brain processes, leading to:

- mood disturbances, including anxiety and depression
- cognitive dysfunction, such as brain fog and memory lapses
- increased risk of neurodegenerative diseases like Alzheimer's and Parkinson's diseases.

The brain's immune system is like a highly trained security force within the command centre, quickly responding to threats with short bursts of inflammation. In a healthy state, this response helps neutralise intruders and repair damage. But chronic inflammation overwhelms neural circuits, disrupts neurotransmitter balance and accelerates cognitive decline.

## The silent mood manipulator

Research has shown that chronic inflammation plays a direct role in mood disorders like depression and anxiety. The reason? Inflammation interferes with neurotransmitter production and dysregulates the body's stress response.

Serotonin and dopamine – your brain's 'feel-good' chemicals – are particularly vulnerable to inflammation. In a healthy system, your body converts the amino acid tryptophan into serotonin, helping to regulate mood. But when inflammation is high, your body diverts tryptophan into kynurenine, a compound that contributes to neurotoxicity rather than emotional balance.

This biochemical hijacking leads to:

- persistent brain fog
- low energy levels
- increased anxiety and depressive symptoms.

Pro-inflammatory cytokines like interleukin-6 and TNF further disrupt neurotransmitter function, trapping you in a cycle of mood imbalances. More than feeling sad or anxious, it's a systemic inflammatory process that reshapes your brain chemistry and emotional resilience.

But where does this inflammation come from? Surprisingly, one of the biggest drivers of brain inflammation isn't even in your brain but in your gut. The gut and brain are in constant communication through the gut–brain axis. When your gut health is compromised, inflammation can spread systemically, affecting your cognitive function, mood and even long-term brain health.

## THE GUT–BRAIN AXIS: How your stomach affects your headspace

Beyond its role in digestion and immune function, the gut plays a profound role in mental health. The connection between the gut and brain, known as the gut–brain axis, is a two-way communication system that influences everything from mood to cognitive function. Emerging research shows that gut bacteria produce neurotransmitters and metabolites that directly impact the brain, shaping emotional stability and neurological resilience.

## GUT MICROBES: The unsung heroes (or villains) of your brain health

Chronic gut inflammation has been associated with anxiety, depression, brain fog and cognitive decline. The gut microbiome influences mental health in several ways:

- **Gut bacteria influence the production and regulation of key neurotransmitter**s like serotonin, dopamine and GABA, which affect mood, stress and cognition. They interact closely with the nervous system through the gut–brain axis, modulating signals between the gut and brain to affect mental health and well-being.
- **Beneficial bacteria ferment fibre into short-chain fatty acids** like butyrate, acetate and propionate, which help reduce neuroinflammation and support brain function. They also influence the production of

brain-derived neurotrophic factor, an essential protein for learning, memory and neuroprotection.

- **The vagus nerve** is a direct motorway between the gut and the brain. When you have gut inflammation, signals sent through the vagus nerve can trigger neuroinflammation, contributing to brain fog, anxiety, depression and cognitive decline.

Gut bacteria may also play a role in early neurological development with diet shaping these effects. Imbalances in the microbiome, known as dysbiosis, have been linked to neurodegenerative conditions such as Alzheimer's and Parkinson's diseases. So strengthening and protecting the integrity of the gut lining is crucial to prevent systemic and neuroinflammation.

## THE BRAIN BREAKDOWN: How inflammation fuels neurodegeneration

Your brain is an intricate network of connections, constantly adapting and changing. Neurodegenerative conditions like Alzheimer's and Parkinson's diseases aren't sudden arrivals. They develop gradually – subtle shifts in how your brain processes information, communicates and maintains its vast network of neurons.

Contributing to this process are factors like:

- chronic stress
- poor diet and nutrition
- environmental toxins
- gut dysbiosis
- genetic predispositions
- hormonal imbalances
- lack of sleep
- sedentary lifestyle.

The blood–brain barrier plays a crucial role here. Normally a selective gatekeeper, this barrier becomes more permeable when you have chronic inflammation, allowing inflammatory compounds to slip through and introduce neurotoxic elements into brain tissue. This ongoing inflammation can contribute to the build-up of harmful proteins, such as beta-amyloid plaques in Alzheimer's, which further damage brain cells. They are like microscopic roadblocks, disrupting neural communication and accelerating cellular damage.

## BRAIN FOOD, THE DIET THAT FIGHTS COGNITIVE DECLINE

The brain responds well to dietary and lifestyle interventions, which can help reverse inflammation-driven mood disorders and enhance emotional resilience. Studies suggest that specific diets can either increase or reduce neuroinflammation:

- Diets high in sugar, refined carbohydrates and trans fats have been linked to elevated inflammatory markers and an increased risk of depression and cognitive decline.
- Anti-inflammatory diets, such as the Mediterranean diet that's rich in polyphenols, omega-3 fatty acids and antioxidants, have been shown to reduce inflammation and protect against mood disorders.
- What you eat is not just about physical health; it directly influences mental clarity, emotional stability and cognitive resilience.

### Good nutrition is your brain's best friend

One of the most effective ways to combat neuroinflammation is through an anti-inflammatory diet rich in brain-supporting nutrients. Clinical trials have found that specific foods and nutrients can regulate inflammation and improve mental health:

- **Omega-3 fatty acids** found in wild-caught salmon, linseeds (flaxseeds), walnuts and extra virgin olive oil can reduce inflammation and alleviate depression in individuals with high inflammatory markers.
- **Polyphenols and antioxidants,** abundant in blueberries, spinach and turmeric, act as natural anti-inflammatory agents, protecting the brain from oxidative stress and neurodegeneration.
- **Gut-friendly foods**, such as fermented vegetables, kefir and sauerkraut, promote a healthy microbiome, which helps regulate systemic inflammation and the gut–brain axis.
- **Mediterranean-inspired meals,** such as a quinoa bowl with roasted vegetables, olive oil and turmeric, or wild salmon with leafy greens and walnuts, can help protect brain function and emotional balance.

The beauty of this approach lies in its simplicity. You're not embarking on some exotic nutritional adventure; you're simply choosing foods that have been nourishing human brains for millennia. Your ancestors would be pleased to know that their traditional wisdom has finally caught up with modern science.

## ALZHEIMER'S: The quiet, inflammatory chat among brain cells

Alzheimer's disease is a gradual transformation of how the brain communicates, remembers and functions. While some memory changes are a natural part of ageing, Alzheimer's represents a profound shift that makes recognising loved ones and following conversations increasingly challenging.

At the heart of this condition lies a delicate biological story of inflammation and cellular communication. Microglia – the brain's own immune system cells – normally clear away harmful waste and toxic proteins such as amyloid-beta plaques and tau tangles. These tiny housekeepers maintain the brain's health, keeping neural pathways clean and functional.

But chronic inflammation disrupts this system. Microglia become overwhelmed and less effective. Instead of protecting the brain, they contribute to cellular stress, creating a cascading cycle of neuron damage. The result is that communication between brain cells breaks down, accelerating cognitive decline. Research reveals that higher inflammation levels significantly increase the risk of developing Alzheimer's. So this isn't a story of inevitable decline, but an invitation to proactive brain care.

## BRAIN FOG: Inflammation's hidden cloud over your mind

After my experience with Long Covid, I struggled with mental fatigue, forgetfulness and a frustrating sense of feeling 'off'. It wasn't just ordinary tiredness – my brain felt enveloped in a dense fog, obscuring my ability to focus, recall details or articulate thoughts. My experiences pointed to a deeper underlying issue: persistent inflammation. I write about the effect of inflammation on cognitive function in my book *Nature's Way to Healing: A Long Covid Guide*.

Inflammation targets key brain regions, particularly the prefrontal cortex and hippocampus, which are fundamental to learning, memory and cognitive flexibility. When these neural centres are under stress, neuroplasticity (the brain's remarkable ability to grow and adapt) becomes impaired.

Compounding this challenge is a notable decrease in brain-derived neurotrophic factor, an essential protein for neuronal survival and growth, while oxidative stress accumulates, systematically draining the brain's energy reserves and amplifying mental exhaustion.

Brain fog is increasingly linked to autoimmune diseases and chronic fatigue syndrome. Research links cognitive impairment to systemic inflammation and mitochondrial dysfunction – conditions where cellular energy production falters.

My personal journey of recovery revealed a transformative insight: targeted interventions can dramatically improve cognitive function. Implementing strategic approaches – focusing on anti-inflammatory nutrition, comprehensive gut health support and holistic lifestyle modifications – significantly restored my mental clarity. I cover many of these in the chapters ahead.

## Inflammation's fingerprint on your thoughts and actions

Chronic inflammation extends beyond physical symptoms, significantly impacting behaviour, motivation and emotional well-being. It disrupts the brain's delicate neurochemical balance and affects neurotransmitters like dopamine, which is responsible for motivation and pleasure. When inflammation interferes with dopamine production and transmission, it can lead to anhedonia, a condition where once-enjoyable activities lose their appeal.

The cascading effects of inflammation on mental health can be profound:

- **Neurotransmitters become imbalanced.** Remember those pro-inflammatory cytokines interleukin-6 and TNF? They interfere with serotonin and dopamine production, increasing the risk of mood disorders.
- **Circadian rhythms are disrupted.** Chronic inflammation disrupts the body's natural sleep–wake cycles, reducing melatonin production and increasing the risk of insomnia. Sleep deprivation then elevates stress hormones like cortisol, creating a cycle that exacerbates inflammation.
- **Brain-derived neurotrophic factor is depleted**. This protein is essential for neuroplasticity, the brain's ability to adapt, grow and heal. Chronic inflammation suppresses this protein, making the brain more vulnerable to cognitive decline, mood disorders and neurodegeneration.

## ENERGY CENTRE BREAKDOWN: Inflammation's role in your endocrine system

Hormones are the body's internal traffic controllers, regulating metabolism, stress, immunity and reproductive health. But chronic inflammation hijacks this system, leading to sluggish metabolism, thyroid dysfunction, adrenal fatigue and hormone-driven conditions like insulin resistance and weight gain.

Low-grade, persistent inflammation can scramble hormone production and desensitise hormone receptors, creating a domino effect of metabolic dysfunction. Research links chronic inflammation to polycystic ovary syndrome, correlating it with insulin resistance and metabolic imbalances. Studies also confirm inflammation's role in conditions like type 2 diabetes, autoimmune thyroid disorders and metabolic syndrome, which thrive in an inflamed body system.

## BLOOD GLUCOSE BLOOPERS: An inflammatory roller-coaster ride

Imagine insulin as the key that unlocks cells so glucose can enter and be used for energy. When chronic inflammation jams the locks, insulin loses effectiveness, causing blood glucose levels to soar. This sets the stage for insulin resistance – one of the primary drivers of type 2 diabetes and metabolic syndrome.

Inflammatory cytokines disrupt insulin signalling, while visceral fat (a major source of inflammation) releases compounds that worsen insulin resistance. Meanwhile, the pancreas struggles to keep up, producing more and more insulin to compensate, eventually burning out. But here's the good news: addressing inflammation through diet, movement and stress reduction can restore your insulin sensitivity and prevent long-term metabolic damage.

## THYROID TROUBLE: A disrupted metabolism

The thyroid, your body's metabolic thermostat, is highly sensitive to inflammation. When under attack, metabolism either grinds to a halt (hypothyroidism) or goes into overdrive (hyperthyroidism).

Inflammation also blocks T4 (inactive thyroid hormone) being converted into T3 (the active form), leaving cells energy-starved and struggling to function. Meanwhile autoimmune thyroid disorders like Hashimoto's and Graves' diseases, where the immune system mistakenly attacks thyroid tissue, are exacerbated by chronic inflammation.

The gut–thyroid connection is another factor. Leaky gut and microbiome imbalances can trigger immune responses that inflame the thyroid, worsening symptoms like fatigue, weight gain and mood swings.

## Inflammation and weight gain

In my clinic recently, I met a frustrated corporate executive who had been struggling with stubborn weight gain. Despite following a strict meal plan and hitting the gym five times a week, the scales wouldn't budge. His exasperation was evident as he described how his GP had advised him to 'cut more calories'.

But his body told a different story – the afternoon energy crashes, the persistent cravings after his protein-rich lunch and that stubborn belly fat pointed to something deeper than just diet and exercise.

If weight loss feels impossible despite healthy eating and exercise, the reason could be chronic inflammation. Inflammation-driven hormonal imbalances can:

- increase fat storage, particularly around the abdomen
- disrupt appetite hormones like leptin, making it harder to feel full
- slow metabolism by affecting mitochondrial function and energy production
- trigger cravings and fatigue, making it difficult to stay consistent with healthy habits.

After addressing his inflammation through targeted nutrition and lifestyle changes, not only did his energy improve, but he finally started seeing changes in his waist circumference and weight.

## ADDRESSING THE ROOT CAUSES OF INFLAMMATION

Rebalancing hormones isn't about quick fixes. When you address the root causes of inflammation, hormonal pathways can function as they're meant to, supporting your metabolism, stress resilience and long-term well-being.

**Key strategies to reset hormonal balance:**

- Consume anti-inflammatory foods, prioritising omega-3-rich foods, fibre and antioxidant-packed vegetables.
- Manage stress and reduce cortisol levels with mindfulness, breathwork and movement.
- Support gut health and strengthen the gut lining with fermented foods, probiotics and prebiotics.
- Regulate blood glucose by avoiding processed carbs, balancing meals with protein and including healthy fats.

- Prioritise sleep, improving melatonin production and supporting circadian rhythms to regulate hormone function.

If your hormones feel out of control, inflammation is likely to be at the centre of the storm. Whether it's insulin resistance, thyroid dysfunction or adrenal fatigue, the common denominator is chronic, low-grade inflammation.

## SECURITY SYSTEM SHOWDOWN: From immune protector to antagonist

Your immune system is your body's central security system with trained emergency responders expertly identifying and eliminating threats like bacteria, viruses and toxins. When chronic inflammation disrupts this finely tuned system, your internal security force becomes confused, mistaking healthy tissues for invaders. This confusion forms the foundation of autoimmune diseases, where your body's defence system turns on itself.

### THE USUAL SUSPECTS: Common autoimmune culprits

Autoimmune conditions may manifest differently but all share a common thread: an overactive immune response fuelled by persistent inflammation. Whether it's the joints in rheumatoid arthritis, the nervous system in multiple sclerosis or the gut lining in inflammatory bowel disease, the underlying mechanism is uncontrolled immune activation.

**Rheumatoid arthritis** often starts subtly (morning stiffness, occasional joint pain) but can escalate into widespread inflammation affecting cartilage, bones and even cardiovascular health. Research indicates that people with rheumatoid arthritis often have gut microbiomes with an overabundance of *Prevotella copri*, a bacterium linked to increased inflammation. Scientists have even identified DNA from gut bacteria in the synovial fluid of rheumatoid arthritis patients, suggesting a direct connection between gut microbes and joint inflammation.

**Lupus** is a multitasking troublemaker that can attack the skin, kidneys, brain and heart, leading to unpredictable flare-ups and systemic damage. Recent research has identified four distinct patterns of disease progression in systemic lupus erythematosus, providing valuable insight into personalised treatment strategies.

**Multiple sclerosis** occurs when immune cells attack the protective myelin sheath around nerve fibres, leading to neuroinflammation and progressive neurological decline. Recent studies have highlighted the role of the gut–brain axis in multiple sclerosis, suggesting that gut microbiome imbalances may exacerbate neuroinflammation.

**Inflammatory bowel disease,** including Crohn's disease and ulcerative colitis, results from chronic gut inflammation that damages the intestinal lining. This weakened barrier lets bacterial endotoxins and undigested food particles enter the bloodstream, triggering systemic immune reactions.

## Breaking the cycle

The encouraging news is that despite their differences, autoimmune conditions share inflammation as their core driver. This means that instead of merely suppressing immune activity with medications, addressing inflammation through diet, lifestyle and environmental changes can lead to lasting improvements.

Your holistic approach to immune balance should include consuming anti-inflammatory foods such as omega-3s, antioxidants and gut-supporting fibre; managing stress through mindfulness and adequate rest; and being aware of your environment by reducing your exposure to toxins and food additives.

## The hidden energy thief

Akong with autoimmune disease, unchecked inflammation steadily drains your vitality in unexpected ways. In my clinic, I see this energy drain show up in the business owner who can't make it through afternoon meetings without nodding off, the yoga teacher whose own practice has become exhausting and the parent who feels too drained to play with their children after work.

This fatigue isn't merely about feeling tired. Persistent inflammation disrupts your body's cellular energy factories (mitochondria), increases oxidative stress and keeps your immune system on constant high alert. The result? Your body diverts precious energy to managing inflammation rather than fuelling your daily activities. Whether it's the brain fog that makes simple tasks feel overwhelming, the mid-afternoon crashes that send you reaching for another coffee or the bone-deep exhaustion that makes exercise feel impossible, chronic inflammation can impact every aspect of your well-being.

This is precisely why my MAP approach focuses on reducing inflammation, calming your nervous system and supercharging your cells. Time and time again in my clinic, I've seen how small, consistent changes can add up to significant improvements in quality of life, helping you reclaim your energy, comfort and well-being.

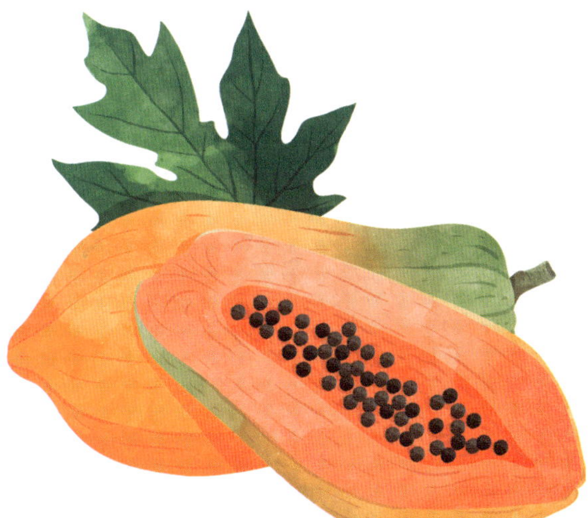

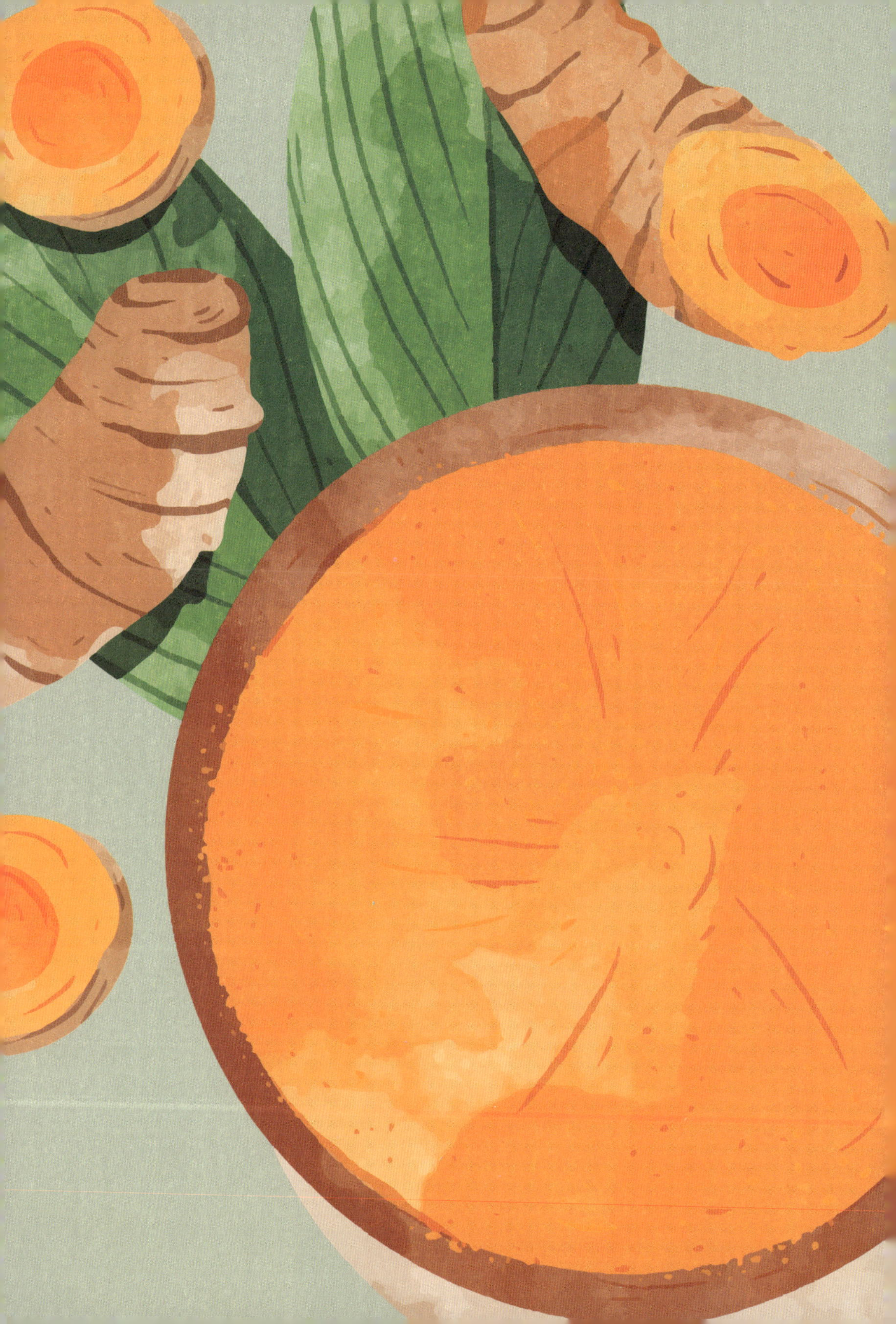

PART 2

# PUTTING OUT THE FIRE

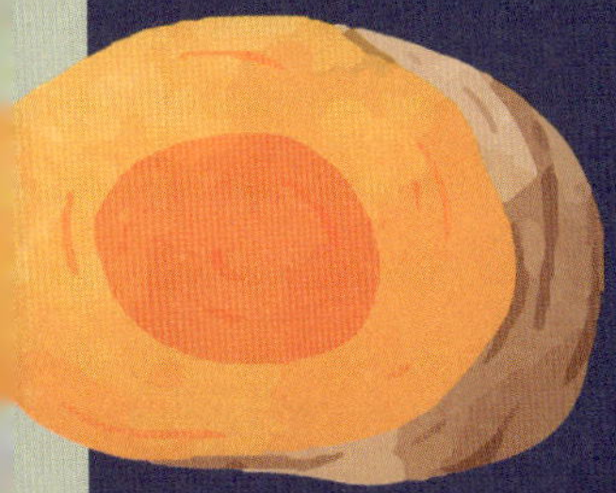

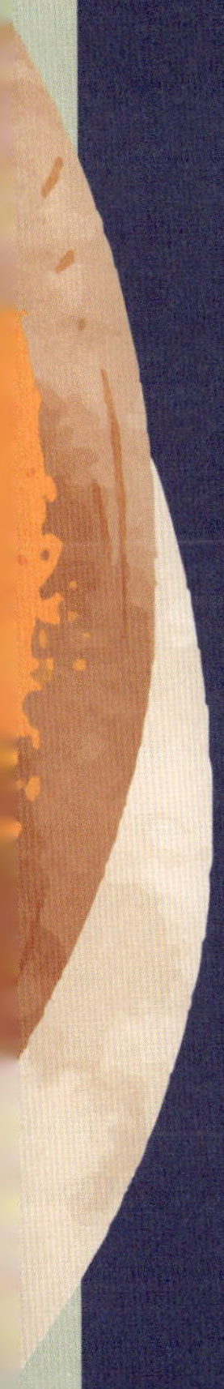

In this part, I'm going to delve into the intricate connections among your gut, mind and overall inflammation, and how the gut is the command centre for your body's immune responses. Imbalances in the gut microbiome can lead to a 'leaky gut', triggering systemic inflammation and contributing to a wide range of chronic health issues. You'll uncover the profound impact of chronic stress and unresolved trauma, which can rewire the gut–brain axis, perpetuating a cycle of inflammation that diet alone cannot fix. Finally, you'll find a comprehensive toolkit of healing strategies that blend ancient wisdom with modern science, offering practical, evidence-based approaches from targeted nutrition to mindful movement and nervous system regulation, so you can restore balance, heal your gut and quench the inflammatory fire.

## CHAPTER 5

# YOUR GUT IS COMMAND CENTRAL

More than just a digestive organ, your gut is the body's command centre for inflammation. Lined with a vast network of immune cells, it continuously surveys everything that enters – food, microbes or toxins – deciding what should be absorbed or eliminated. Communication between the gut and immune system is finely tuned but, when disrupted, it can mistakenly trigger chronic inflammation, fuelling everything from digestive disorders to autoimmune conditions, brain fog and even heart disease.

Bacteria in your gut help regulate inflammation. These microbes produce short-chain fatty acids, which calm immune overactivity and strengthen the intestinal lining. However, when your microbial balance is disrupted – due to poor diet, stress, infections or environmental toxins – the gut barrier can weaken, allowing harmful substances to leak into the bloodstream. Often referred to as 'leaky gut', this phenomenon sets off alarm bells in the immune system, leading to widespread inflammation that can impact nearly every organ in the body.

By understanding these gut–immune mechanisms, we can proactively support our microbiome, repair our gut lining and calm the inflammatory storm before it becomes chronic.

**How do you know if you have gut issues?** You might feel tired or experience pain after eating, suffer from bloating, or have dysregulated bowel movements like constipation or diarrhoea. If this sounds familiar, the five-step approach in this chapter is your starting point.

## HOW GUT BACTERIA INFLUENCE INFLAMMATION

The human gut is a thriving ecosystem home to trillions of microorganisms – bacteria, viruses, fungi and archaea – collectively known as the gut microbiome. Along with aiding digestion, these microorganisms work together to maintain balance, shaping immune responses and influencing inflammation.

## GUT BACTERIA: The immune system's secret weapon

Your immune system has most of its security detail (about 70%–80%) strategically positioned in the gut. Here, these vigilant emergency response workers work closely with gut-associated lymphoid tissue, a specialised network that's like a surveillance system. In the security control room, microbial activity is monitored and decisions made about when to raise the alarm are being made.

Beneficial gut bacteria are like expert security consultants for this internal protection team. They help train your immune system, fine-tuning its ability to distinguish between welcome guests and actual intruders. Certain bacterial allies, such as *Faecalibacterium prausnitzii*, act like peacekeepers, producing anti-inflammatory compounds that help maintain order. Meanwhile, other beneficial bacteria prevent troublemakers like *E. coli* and *Klebsiella pneumoniae* from gaining a foothold.

## INFLAMMATORY SIGNALS: When your microbiome sends SOS messages

The gut microbiome regulates your body's inflammatory processes. Beneficial bacteria produce a range of anti-inflammatory compounds, particularly short-chain fatty acids. These molecular peacekeepers calm immune responses, strengthen your gut barrier, power the cells that line your intestines, and even influence your metabolism and mineral absorption.

Your gut lining (the epithelial barrier) is like a highly sophisticated security fence around your most valuable property. It's just one cell thick but is remarkably effective when working properly. The cells are held together by special proteins (tight junctions) that are like security gates, allowing in beneficial nutrients while keeping out harmful substances.

When your gut microbiome becomes imbalanced (when we consume processed foods, are stressed, have taken antibiotics or been exposed to environmental toxins), troublemaking bacteria can gain the upper hand. They produce lipopolysaccharides (LPS) – toxic compounds that trigger widespread inflammation. These bacterial toxins ring alarm bells in your immune system.

Elevated serum LPS levels are significantly correlated with increased production of the inflammatory markers CRP, interleukin-6 and TNF.

Here's what happens next:

- These bacterial toxins slip through the weakened epithelial barrier.
- The immune system identifies them as threats and launches a response.
- This response triggers inflammation, which further damages the gut lining.

As the cycle continues, more toxins can escape and systemic inflammation worsens. While LPS itself isn't found in food, our dietary choices can influence its production:

- Highly processed foods feed harmful bacteria, increasing LPS production.
- Excess saturated fats can help LPS cross the gut barrier more easily.
- High-sugar diets promote the growth of LPS-producing bacteria.

## When things go sideways

When the gut lining becomes compromised, bacterial toxins, undigested food particles and inflammatory by-products like LPS can enter the bloodstream, triggering immune activation and widespread inflammation. Once these inflammatory molecules enter circulation, they don't stay confined to your gut – they travel throughout your body like troublemakers spreading chaos. To better understand this process, the following sequence illustrates how gut imbalances escalate into systemic inflammation and affect multiple body systems.

## LEAKY GUT, LEAKY LIFE: The inflammation trigger you didn't see coming

Once harmful substances escape the gut, the immune system detects them as threats and initiates an inflammatory response. This leads to the release of inflammatory cytokines interleukin-6, TNF and CRP.

While acute inflammation is a natural defence mechanism, chronic immune activation can result in widespread systemic inflammation.

### GUT BACTERIA IMBALANCE (DYSBIOSIS)

**Beneficial bacteria decline while harmful microbes multiply.**
Barrier breakdown

↓

**The gut lining weakens, allowing toxins through.**
Leaky gut syndrome

↓

**Bacterial toxins like LPS enter circulation.**
Immune activation

↓

**The immune system responds by releasing inflammatory cytokines.**
Systemic inflammation

↓

**Persistent inflammation contributes to chronic disease risk.**

Leaky gut has been linked to numerous disorders:

- **Autoimmune diseases** such as rheumatoid arthritis, lupus and Hashimoto's thyroiditis
- **Metabolic disorders** such as insulin resistance, type 2 diabetes and obesity
- **Neurological conditions** such as depression, anxiety, brain fog and neurodegenerative diseases
- **Digestive disorders** such as irritable bowel syndrome (IBS), Crohn's disease and ulcerative colitis

One of the most common complaints I see in my clinic is unexplained fatigue, bloating and difficulty digesting certain foods. Many clients have been told they just need to 'eat clean' or take probiotics, yet their symptoms persist. In nearly every case, gut permeability is at the root of the issue.

When we address leaky gut, inflammation levels drop, digestion improves and symptoms start to resolve. The gut lining is highly regenerative, renewing itself every few days, meaning that with the right support, it can heal and restore its protective function.

### STEPS TO PATCH UP YOUR LEAKY GUT

- **Remove inflammatory triggers.** Reduce processed foods, refined sugar, gluten, dairy (if sensitive), excessive alcohol and artificial additives – these weaken the gut lining.
- **Nourish the gut lining.** Consume healing foods such as bone broth, omega-3-rich foods, polyphenols and collagen-boosting nutrients to repair intestinal integrity.
- **Repopulate with probiotics and prebiotics.** Eat probiotic fermented foods like fermented vegetables and kefir, while feeding gut bacteria with prebiotic fibres found in garlic, onions and asparagus.
- **Increase fibre intake.** Support digestion and gut flora with a mix of soluble fibre (chia seeds, oats, legumes), insoluble fibre (vegetables, whole grains) and resistant starch (green bananas, cooked then cooled potatoes).
- **Manage stress and improve sleep.** Reduce gut-disrupting stress through mindfulness, deep breathing and ensuring quality sleep to maintain microbiome balance.

## REPAIR STARTS HERE: The four step gut-healing reset

As I explained in my book *Heal Your Gut*, the gut microbiome has the complexity of the Amazon rainforest. Just as the rainforest thrives through intricate relationships among countless species – from towering trees to tiny insects – your gut houses millions of microorganisms working in harmony. When this internal ecosystem maintains its rich diversity, it creates a robust defence system that keeps inflammation in check.

However, just as deforestation can devastate a rainforest's delicate balance, various factors can reduce diversity in your microbiota. This loss of beneficial bacteria has been linked to numerous chronic conditions, from obesity and depression to autoimmune diseases and inflammatory bowel disease.

Healing the gut isn't about quick fixes or restrictive cleanses – it's about long-term nourishment. If the gut lining is weakened and gut bacteria are imbalanced, the body cannot properly absorb nutrients or regulate inflammation. Jumping straight into an anti-inflammatory diet without first addressing gut imbalances often leads to limited benefits. Many clients have tried anti-inflammatory diets but still struggle with digestive issues, food sensitivities or fatigue. If you feel tired or experience pain after eating, bloating or dysregulated bowel movements, here's what I recommend:

## Step 1. Remove inflammatory triggers

- Refined sugars and processed foods feed harmful bacteria, promoting dysbiosis.
- Gluten increases zonulin levels, which loosens tight junctions in the gut lining.
- Excess alcohol, antibiotics and non-steroidal anti-inflammatory drugs (NSAIDs) like ibuprofen weaken gut barrier integrity. Artificial sweeteners including aspartame, saccharin, sucralose and acesulfame potassium (Ace-K) reduce beneficial bacteria such as *Lactobacillus* and *Bifidobacterium*.
- Industrial seed oils (soybean, corn, canola) promote inflammation.

## Step 2. Nourish the gut lining with healing foods

- Bone broth provides collagen, gelatine and glutamine for intestinal barrier integrity.
- Omega-3 fatty acids found in wild-caught fish, linseeds (flaxseeds) and walnuts regulate inflammation.
- Polyphenol-rich foods such as berries, green tea and extra virgin olive oil support microbial balance.
- L-glutamine found in cabbage, spinach and eggs aids gut cellular repair.

- Zinc and vitamin A found in oysters, sweet potatoes and carrots strengthen the gut lining.

### Step 3. Restore balance with probiotics and prebiotics

- Probiotic-rich foods like sauerkraut, Greek yogurt, cultured cheese, fermented olives, kefir and fermented vegetables introduce beneficial bacteria.
- Prebiotic fibre found in garlic, onions, leeks and asparagus fuel beneficial microbes.
- Resistant starch from green bananas and cooked, cooled rice produces short-chain fatty acids essential for gut repair.
- Research shows prebiotic fibres selectively nourish beneficial bacteria like *Bifidobacteria* and *Akkermansia*, which maintain gut barrier integrity and regulate inflammation.

### Step 4. Increase fibre for a healthy microbiome

- Soluble fibre (oats, chia seeds, legumes) feeds beneficial bacteria.
- Insoluble fibre (vegetables, whole grains) promotes healthy digestion.
- Resistant starch supports gut barrier function and short-chain fatty acid production.

## GUT HEALTH SUPERCHARGED SUPERSTARS: Foods to supercharge your gut

Your gut bacteria thrive on two key dietary components: fibre and polyphenols. Think of fibre as the building blocks and polyphenols as the premium fuel that helps your beneficial bacteria flourish.

### Breakfast champions

- Add ground linseeds (flaxseeds) and berries to your porridge for soluble fibre and polyphenols.
- Blend chia seeds and cacao powder into your smoothie.
- Swap regular tea for green tea or matcha.
- Top yogurt with pomegranate seeds and oats.

### Lunch and dinner boosters

- Start with a base of legumes and drizzle with extra virgin olive oil.
- Add red or purple onions to salads.
- Include plenty of leafy greens.
- Season generously with turmeric and freshly ground black pepper.

### Smart snacking

- Choose dark chocolate (85% or higher) with berries.
- Mix chia seeds into yogurt.
- Snack on hummus with sardine crackers.

## THE FOUNDATION FOR LASTING HEALTH

By healing your gut, you're laying the groundwork for vibrant health. By removing inflammatory triggers, nourishing the gut lining, restoring microbial balance and managing stress, you create optimal conditions for reduced inflammation and improved health. Your gut isn't just for digestion, it's your body's inflammation control centre. Master your gut health, and you'll discover the profound impact it has on every aspect of your well-being.

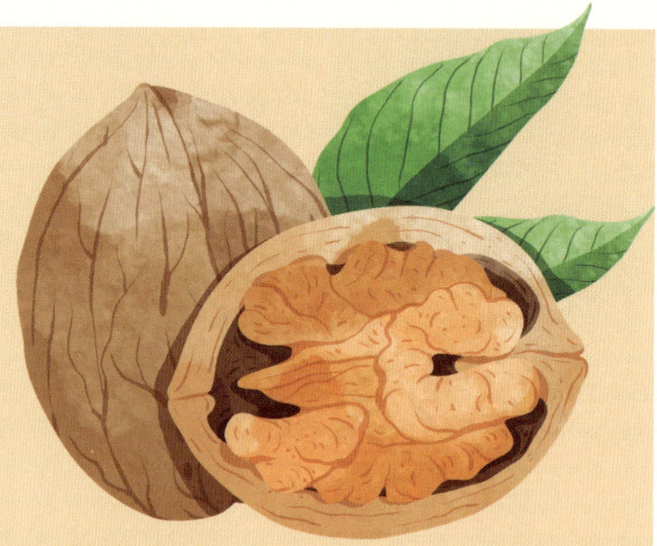

CHAPTER 6

# YOUR MIND–BODY CONNECTION: HEALING TRAUMA AND STRESS

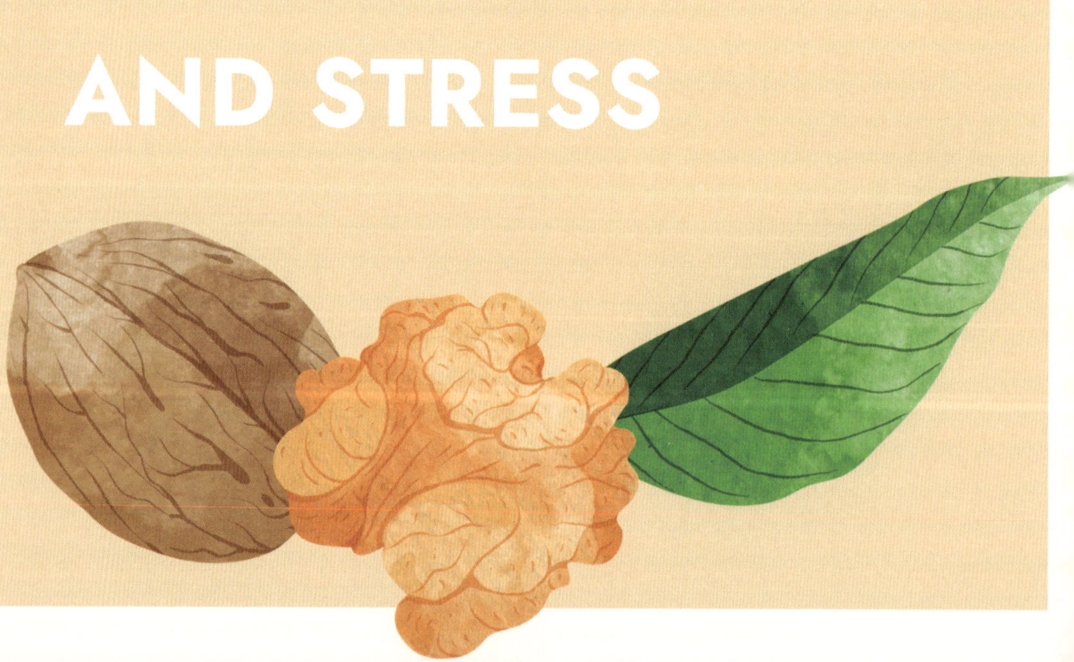

In Chapter 5 we explored how gut dysfunction triggers inflammation throughout your body and how to reset your gut. But another powerful force can hijack this entire system: unresolved trauma and chronic stress rewire the communication pathways between your gut and brain. This rewiring triggers inflammation through disrupted neural pathways, compromised barriers and dysregulated immune responses, and it needs mind–body healing.

## THE MIND–BODY CONNECTION: Where trauma meets stress

Trauma and chronic stress are forms of nervous system dysregulation that fundamentally alter how your body perceives and responds to threats. While we often think of trauma as singular events and stress as daily pressures, they're interconnected. Trauma is a form of chronic stress that rewrites your body's operating system. Whether you're dealing with unresolved trauma from the past or persistent stress in the present, they create the same inflammatory cascade through your nervous system, gut and immune function. To heal, you need to address the root nervous system dysfunction, not just manage symptoms.

Your nervous system is designed to protect your physical home. When it's functioning properly, it can distinguish between someone delivering a package and a genuine intruder. But trauma and chronic stress are like having that alarm system permanently stuck on 'alert' – even a cat walking past becomes a five-alarm emergency. Your body's brilliant survival mechanisms, designed to keep you safe during genuine danger, become the thing that keeps you chronically inflamed and unwell.

Unlike diet or environmental factors that come and go, trauma and chronic stress operate differently. Think of it like the difference between a brief power surge that flickers your lights versus a lightning strike that blows your entire electrical system. Traumatic and stressful experiences don't just trigger inflammation; they fundamentally alter how your body perceives safety, creating a heightened inflammatory baseline that affects every aspect of your health.

The reason I'm dedicating a chapter to this isn't to pathologise your experiences, but to acknowledge that healing happens in layers. You might have the cleanest diet in the world, take every supplement known to humanity and still feel rubbish because your nervous system is trying to run the latest software on a computer that's still operating on Windows 95.

## THE EVOLUTIONARY PERSPECTIVE: When ancient wiring meets modern life

Our nervous systems evolved magnificently for acute, short-term threats – the kind where you either escaped the sabre-toothed tiger or became its lunch. The problem is that our modern lives are full of chronic, low-grade stressors that our ancient wiring interprets as ongoing threats. Your nervous system can't tell the difference between a predator chasing you and your boss sending passive-aggressive emails at 11 pm.

When the vagus nerve, our body's primary 'rest and digest' pathway, becomes chronically active the message to calm down and heal gets lost in the static. Meanwhile, inflammatory cytokines, which should be temporary messengers calling for help, set up permanent camp in your tissues.

This chronic stress response taxes your nervous system and immune function, increasing vulnerability to anxiety, depression and digestive disorders. Understanding this evolutionary mismatch is key to developing mind–body healing strategies that restore balance and resilience.

## THE VAGUS NERVE: YOUR BODY'S INFORMATION SUPERHIGHWAY

The vagus nerve is essentially your body's information superhighway between the brain and gut. This cranial nerve carries 80% of the signals from gut to brain, making it the primary communication channel in the gut–brain axis.

Being chronically stressed compromises this nerve's strength and effectiveness, or vagal tone. Think of it like internet bandwidth: when it's working well, information flows smoothly in both directions. But stress is like having multiple people streaming Netflix while running video calls – everything slows down and communication becomes unreliable.

Reduced vagal tone is associated with increased inflammatory markers, poor digestive function and decreased heart rate variability. It's measurable too – heart rate variability is a real-time indicator of vagal tone and nervous system resilience.

## How trauma and stress rewire your brain

At its core, trauma and chronic stress reshape your brain's architecture through three key players:

- The amygdala (threat detector) becomes hypervigilant, constantly scanning for danger.
- The hippocampus (memory processor) shrinks, making it harder to distinguish between past dangers and present safety.
- The prefrontal cortex (regulation centre) weakens, making it difficult to calm fear responses.

This disruption floods the body with cortisol, keeping the stress response on high alert. Over time this exhausts the immune system, weakens the gut barrier and increases inflammation. The balance of serotonin and dopamine is also disrupted, leading to emotional numbness or an increased need for stimulation.

For someone carrying unresolved trauma or chronic stress, their nervous system's alarm bells go off at the slightest touch – whether it's a minor disagreement, unexpected noise or subtle shift in a loved one's tone. The sympathetic nervous system keeps you in perpetual fight-or-flight mode, while your vagus nerve is less effective at hitting the brakes.

### The neurochemical cascade

When your stress response activates, it's like dominoes falling. First, your hypothalamus releases corticotropin-releasing hormone, which signals your pituitary gland to produce adrenocorticotropic hormone (ACTH). This then tells your adrenal glands to pump out cortisol and adrenaline. In acute situations, this cascade is brilliant – it mobilises energy, heightens your awareness and prepares you for action.

But when this system runs continuously, it's like having your car's engine redlining 24/7. The cortisol that normally spikes then returns to baseline remains persistently elevated, leading to what researchers call 'cortisol dysregulation'. This doesn't just mean too much cortisol, it can also mean too little as exhausted adrenal glands struggle to meet constant demands.

The consequences are profound. Chronic cortisol elevation increases the pro-inflammatory cytokines interleukin-6, TNF and CRP. These are designed to coordinate healing responses, but when they are constantly elevated, they become the problem rather than the solution and a key driver for inflammation.

## THE GUT–BRAIN CONNECTION UNDER SIEGE

The gut–brain connection is vulnerable to chronic stress and trauma. Research shows individuals with adverse childhood experiences are twice as likely to develop IBS, demonstrating the deep biological imprinting of these experiences.

When trauma enters this delicate system, particularly during early life, it causes the vagus nerve to lose its ability to regulate inflammation and maintain healthy gut function. This disruption cascades through multiple biological systems, particularly the immune system:

- **The microbiome is disrupted.** Chronic stress decimates beneficial bacteria while allowing harmful species to proliferate, reducing diversity and weakening immune responses. Studies show that chronic stress can reduce beneficial *Lactobacillus* and *Bifidobacterium* populations by up to 50%, while pathogenic bacteria like *Clostridium* and *Enterobacter* simultaneously increase.
- **Gut permeability increases.** The gut lining transforms from an impenetrable fortress to a porous membrane in chronic stress. The tight junction proteins that normally seal the intestinal barrier (including claudin-1, occludin and zonula occludens-1) become compromised under chronic stress. As unwanted molecules penetrate the intestinal barrier, the immune system mobilises, releasing inflammatory cytokines that create a self-perpetuating cycle.
- **Gut rhythm becomes erratic.** The enteric nervous system becomes dysregulated, creating erratic digestive movements, alternating between rapid transit and prolonged stagnation that manifest as IBS-like symptoms. The migrating motor complex, which normally sweeps through the intestines like a biological housekeeper, becomes irregular and ineffective.
- **The gut becomes more sensitive.** Trauma rewrites the brain's interpretation of gut signals, making normal digestive processes feel amplified and uncomfortable. The gut's sensory neurons become hyperexcitable, making routine digestion an uncomfortable experience.

# CASE STUDY: SARAH'S AUTOIMMUNE JOURNEY

| CLIENT PROFILE |
|---|
| Sarah, 36, yoga teacher with Hashimoto's thyroiditis |
| **Primary symptoms**<br>Debilitating fatigue, joint pain, bloating, constipation, anxiety |
| **The paradox**<br>Despite years of clean eating, movement and mindfulness practices, her autoimmune flares persisted. |
| **The hidden struggle**<br>Pushing through exhaustion to maintain her 'healthy' image, Sarah believed more discipline would finally heal her body. |

## The deeper story

Sarah had spent years dedicated to wellness practices, yet she still suffered from symptoms that left her feeling frustrated and betrayed by her own body. As a yoga teacher, she felt immense pressure to embody radiant health. When students complimented her on her glow, she'd smile while hiding the joint pain that made simple poses agony. When colleagues discussed their latest cleanse, she'd nod enthusiastically and secretly plan an even more restrictive protocol.

Her Instagram feed showed perfectly arranged smoothie bowls and challenging yoga poses, but behind the camera, she was exhausted, bloated and increasingly anxious about every symptom. She'd wake at 5 am for meditation, push through a demanding yoga practice, sip her green juice and smile through teaching six classes – all while her body screamed for rest.

## The trauma–immune connection

Sarah revealed she had spent years in an emotionally abusive relationship during her twenties. Though she had left the relationship 5 years prior, she carried deep self-criticism that had transformed into perfectionism in health and wellness. Her ex-partner's voice had become her inner critic: *You're not doing enough. You're weak. You need to try harder.*

The unprocessed emotions from her past relationship kept her nervous system in mild fight-or-flight mode, triggering chronic inflammation. This inflammation was worsened by increased gut permeability, which contributed to ongoing autoimmune activity, while her relentless inner critic kept her body's cortisol levels elevated, suppressing healthy immune regulation.

Sarah's case illustrates a common pattern: when healing becomes another source of stress. She'd turned her health journey into a performance, complete with rigid rules, self-criticism when she 'slipped up' and anxiety about every symptom. Her nervous system couldn't differentiate between genuine threats and her own internal pressure to be the 'perfect' wellness practitioner.

## The healing process

We focused on self-compassion as a physiological intervention rather than restricting her diet further. Sarah worked on reframing her negative self-talk, shifting from *I need to be more disciplined* to *I deserve to rest.* She practised self-compassion meditations, which research shows can reduce inflammatory markers by up to 25%.

The breakthrough moment came during one session, when Sarah admitted she spoke to herself more harshly than she'd ever speak to a student. We practised her responding to physical discomfort with the same gentle encouragement she'd offer someone in her yoga class. This simple shift began rewiring her stress response.

Sarah started incorporating vocal work to regulate her vagus nerve. She began humming while preparing meals, singing in the car and incorporating toning exercises (like long exhalations with sound) into her personal practice. These simple interventions increased her body's ability to switch out of stress mode.

Sarah noticed her digestion improved dramatically on days she sang or hummed regularly. Her body was literally vibrating itself back to balance.

## Movement as play, not performance

Instead of pushing through advanced yoga postures, Sarah embraced gentle, restorative yoga and intuitive movement. She listened to her body's cues instead of overriding them. Some days, this meant child's pose instead of headstand. Other days, it meant a gentle walk instead of a vigorous flow.

Sarah began offering 'Gentle Yoga for Sensitive Bodies' classes, which became her most popular sessions. Teaching from her authentic experience rather than perceived perfection created deeper connection with her students.

## Nervous system nutrition

We introduced the 'eat to heal' approach by adding gut-soothing foods alongside nervous system support. Warm, nourishing foods like soups, stews and lightly cooked vegetables replaced raw, restrictive diets. Magnesium-rich foods, targeted probiotics and adaptogenic herbs supported her stress resilience.

Sarah discovered that her body responded better to warm, cooked foods than the raw salads she'd been forcing herself to eat. Her bloating decreased and her energy stabilised when she honoured her body's actual needs rather than following rigid rules.

| THE RESULTS<br>Within 6 weeks, remarkable changes emerged. |
|---|
| **Digestive symptoms**<br>Bloating eased significantly, and constipation resolved |
| **Energy levels**<br>Sustainable energy throughout the day – no more afternoon crashes |
| **Autoimmune markers**<br>Thyroid antibodies decreased, inflammatory markers improved |
| **Mental clarity**<br>Reduced anxiety, and improved focus and decision-making |
| **Relationship with her body**<br>Shifted from frustration to appreciation |

## The deeper transformation

Sarah's transformation wasn't about adding more healing modalities but changing her relationship with healing itself. She discovered her body responded better to gentle consistency than intense perfectionism. The chronic inflammation that had plagued her for years began to subside as Sarah released self-judgement and supported her nervous system.

'I spent years trying to heal my body by fighting it,' Sarah reflects. 'Real healing happened when I started listening to it instead. My autoimmune condition taught me that sometimes the most radical thing you can do is be kind to yourself.'

## Key insights for practice

- **Perfectionism is inflammatory.** The stress of trying to be the 'perfect' healthy person can perpetuate the very symptoms we're trying to heal.
- **Self-compassion is physiological.** Gentle self-talk measurably reduces inflammatory markers.
- **The nervous system needs safety.** Healing happens in a state of calm, not stress.
- **Movement quality matters more than intensity.** Gentle, consistent movement often outperforms intense, sporadic exercise for autoimmune conditions.
- **Food relationships matter.** How we think about food affects how our body processes it.

Sarah's story reminds that, for healing, we often need to examine not just what we're doing, but how we're being while we're doing it. Sometimes the most powerful medicine is the permission to rest, be imperfect and trust our body's wisdom rather than override it with our mind's demands.

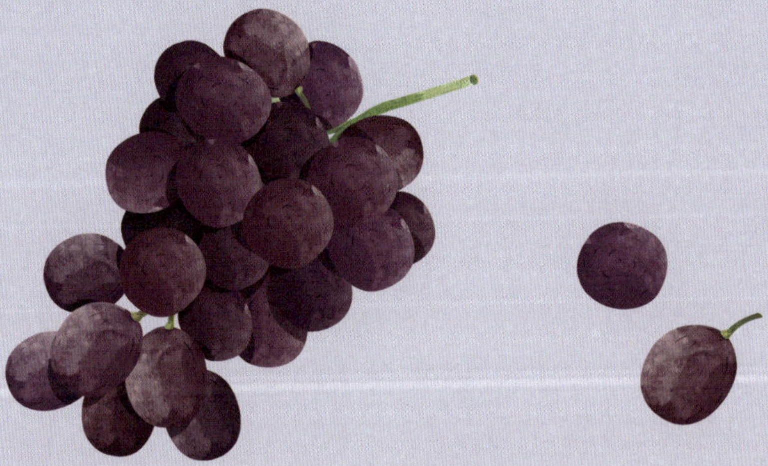

## THE GENERATIONAL IMPACT: When trauma echoes through time

Childhood trauma doesn't just leave difficult memories, it alters the body's operating system. Early experiences shape the body's gene expression, immune responses and nervous system regulation. Research shows that adults who experienced childhood trauma often have higher levels of the inflammatory markers interleukin-6, TNF and CRP even decades later.

Perhaps most remarkably, scientists have observed that trauma can influence future generations through epigenetic changes – modifications to gene expression that can be passed down without altering the DNA sequence itself. This has been documented in descendants of Holocaust survivors and communities affected by war and famine, where the biological impacts of trauma can echo through generations.

Our bodies are not separate from our histories. Every experience, from minor stress to deep trauma, leaves an imprint. Some of these imprints fade, while others become deeply embedded, manifesting as chronic pain, digestive disorders or persistent fatigue.

To understand how profoundly trauma affects our biology and psyche, it's important to explore how early experiences shape not only our memories but also the complex interplay among the gut, brain, immune and nervous system. These create biological and behavioural patterns that can echo across generations and last long after the original events, but we can learn how to undo them.

## HEALING APPROACHES: Rewiring your system

The same neuroplasticity that allowed trauma and stress to imprint itself can become your greatest ally in healing. Here are evidence-based approaches to restore balance and calm the nervous system.

# SOMATIC HEALING: Working with the body's wisdom

Traditional talk therapy, while extremely valuable, often doesn't address the body's stored responses to trauma. Somatic approaches work directly with the nervous system's physical responses:

- **Somatic experiencing** helps interrupted survival responses to complete, allowing trapped traumatic energy to discharge naturally. It's like giving your nervous system permission to finish what it started. Practitioners guide clients through gentle awareness of physical sensations, helping the body complete thwarted defensive responses.
- **Eye movement desensitisation and reprocessing** uses bilateral stimulation to help your brain to process traumatic memories as past events, reducing their capacity to trigger stress responses. The rhythmic eye movements or alternating tactile stimulation helps integrate traumatic memories into normal memory networks.
- **Breathwork and mindfulness** such as coherent breathing (5 seconds in, 5 seconds out) rapidly shifts your nervous system from stress to relaxation, reducing inflammatory markers and improving immune function. This specific rhythm activates the baroreflex, which helps regulate blood pressure and heart rate variability.
- **Polyvagal-informed practices** such as gentle neck work, vocal exercises and rhythmic movements directly engage the vagus nerve, helping to regulate your nervous system's response to stress. These practices are based on Dr Stephen Porges's polyvagal theory, which explains how our autonomic nervous system evolved to detect safety and threat.

## THE POLYVAGAL THEORY: A roadmap to regulation

Dr Porges's polyvagal theory provides a brilliant framework for understanding nervous system responses. According to this theory, we have three main states:

- **Ventral vagal** (social engagement) is your optimal state where you feel safe, connected, and capable of rest and digest functions. Your heart rate variability is high, inflammation is low, and healing happens naturally.
- **Sympathetic** (fight/flight) system activates when the body detects a threat to mobilise energy for action. Your heart rate increases, breathing becomes shallow and non-essential functions like digestion shut down.
- **Dorsal vagal** (collapse/freeze) system activates when a threat is overwhelming or escape seems impossible, leading to shutdown, disconnection and conservation of energy.

Understanding these states helps explain why the traditional 'just relax' advice often fails. If your nervous system is stuck in sympathetic activation or dorsal collapse, you can't simply think your way into ventral vagal safety. You need to work with the body's wisdom to shift states.

## MINDFULNESS: Your nervous system's reset button

Mindfulness and breathing practices serve as gentle instructors for your nervous system. Each conscious breath is like pressing the reset button, signalling your body to shift from high alert into calm. When you meditate regularly, you're training your vagus nerve (your body's natural anti-inflammatory pathway) to respond more effectively.

Research backs this up beautifully. Regular mindfulness practitioners show measurably lower levels of inflammatory markers in their blood. The beauty of mindfulness lies in its variety – each practice offers a different way to interrupt the conversation between stress and inflammation, helping your body remember its natural state of balance.

Experiment with these evidence-based practices to find what resonates most with your body and lifestyle:

- **Mindfulness meditation** reduces cortisol levels and decreases amygdala activity. Start with 5 minutes daily of following your breath. Research shows that regular mindfulness practice changes your brain's structure, increasing grey matter in areas associated with emotional regulation while decreasing activity in the amygdala.
- **Loving-kindness meditation** cultivates self-compassion, reduces social isolation and improves immune function. This practice involves systematically sending wishes of well-being to yourself, loved ones, neutral people, difficult people and all beings.
- **Body scanning** brings your awareness to physical sensations, helping you recognise and release stored tension. This practice helps develop interoceptive awareness (your ability to sense internal body signals), which is often compromised by trauma and chronic stress.

## THE NEUROSCIENCE OF MINDFULNESS

Brain imaging studies reveal that mindfulness practices create measurable changes in brain structure and function. The prefrontal cortex, which is responsible for executive function and emotional regulation, becomes more active and develops stronger connections to the amygdala, essentially giving you better brakes on your stress response.

Meanwhile, the default mode network (the brain's screensaver that often runs negative thought loops) becomes less active. This is significant because overactivity in the default mode network is associated with rumination, anxiety and depression.

## Sound and vibration healing

Specific frequencies can alter your brainwave activity and reduce stress-induced inflammation:

- **Therapeutic frequencies** such as 432 Hz and 528 Hz help reduce inflammatory cytokines. Try listening to these frequencies on streaming platforms or apps. They are thought to promote cellular repair and reduce stress hormones, though the mechanisms are still being researched.
- **Vocal practices** such as humming, chanting or extended vocal sounds create vibrations that directly stimulate the vagus nerve. The act of humming creates nitric oxide, a vasodilator that improves circulation and has anti-inflammatory properties.
- **Sound baths** are immersive experiences with singing bowls and gongs. They activate the parasympathetic nervous system. The complex harmonics and vibrations help train brainwaves into more relaxed states.

### THE VIBRATIONAL MEDICINE PERSPECTIVE

Every cell in your body vibrates at specific frequencies, and chronic stress can disrupt these natural oscillations. Sound healing works by providing external frequencies that help restore cellular harmony. It's like tuning an instrument – when one string is out of tune, it affects the whole orchestra.

The vagus nerve is especially responsive to vibration, which helps explain why humming, singing and chanting have been used as healing practices across cultures for millennia. Modern research confirms what traditional healers have long known: sound can be medicine.

# NATURE'S PHARMACY: The biophilia effect

Humans have an innate affinity for nature, termed 'biophilia' by biologist E.O. Wilson. Exposure to natural environments consistently reduces cortisol, lowers blood pressure and improves mood. Even viewing nature through windows or looking at nature photography can provide measurable benefits.

The fractal patterns found in nature, from tree branches to cloud formations, have been shown to reduce physiological stress. It's as if our nervous systems are calibrated to find peace in the organic, irregular patterns of the natural world rather than the geometric rigidity of urban environments.

Try these practices to reduce stress:

- **Forest bathing** by engaging all senses in nature reduces cortisol, enhances immune function and improves mood. The Japanese practice of shinrin-yoku involves mindful immersion in forest environments, which has been shown to increase natural killer cell activity and reduce inflammatory markers.
- **Grounding** by having direct contact with earth's surface (walking barefoot) can reduce inflammation and normalise circadian rhythms. The earth's surface carries a negative electrical charge; direct contact helps neutralise the positive charge that accumulates from chronic stress and electromagnetic exposure.
- **Garden therapy** by caring for plants provides mindful movement and connection with natural growth cycles. The act of nurturing plants mirrors the process of nurturing yourself, while soil microbes have been shown to have antidepressant effects.

## MOVEMENT AS MEDICINE

**Walking meditation**

Slow, deliberate walking creates a moving meditation that interrupts racing thoughts. The bilateral nature of walking naturally activates both brain hemispheres, promoting integration and calm.

**Gentle strength training**

Compound movements and bodyweight exercises build resilience without excessive inflammatory stress. The key is finding the sweet spot where you challenge your body enough to promote adaptation without triggering excessive stress hormones.

**Mobility work**

Joint rotations and stretches maintain synovial fluid health and reduce inflammatory accumulation. Gentle movement helps circulate lymphatic fluid, which carries inflammatory debris away from tissues.

## Exercise as nervous system training

The right type of exercise can serve as nervous system training, helping you practice moving between activation and recovery. High-intensity exercise temporarily increases stress hormones, but if followed by adequate recovery, it can improve your body's ability to return to baseline – essentially training your nervous system to be more resilient.

The key is avoiding the trap of using exercise as another stressor. If you're already chronically stressed, adding intense exercise can be counterproductive. Instead, focus on movement that feels nourishing and helps you connect with your body.

## VAGUS NERVE PRACTICES: Your direct line to calm

These practices activate your vagus nerve to calm your nervous system:

- **Humming** creates vibrations that stimulate the vagus nerve. Try 3–5 minutes of continuous humming. The vibrations travel through your chest and throat, directly stimulating vagal pathways.
- **Coherent breathing** with equal inhalations and exhalations (5 seconds each) rapidly shifts your system from stress to relaxation. This specific rhythm maximises heart rate variability and activates the baroreflex.
- **Give yourself a butterfly hug** by crossing arms over chest, hands on opposite shoulders and gently tapping alternating sides. This bilateral stimulation activates the parasympathetic nervous system within minutes.
- **Cold exposure** with brief cold showers or ice baths can stimulate the vagus nerve and improve your stress resilience. Start with 30 seconds of cold water at the end of your shower and gradually increase duration.

### ADVANCED VAGAL PRACTICES

**Gargling**

Vigorous gargling activates the muscles in the back of your throat, which are innervated by the vagus nerve. Try gargling for 30 seconds several times daily.

**Singing**

The act of singing, especially in groups, is one of the most powerful vagal stimulators. The combination of controlled breathing, vocal vibration and social connection creates a perfect storm of nervous system regulation.

**Laughter**

Genuine laughter activates the vagus nerve through rhythmic breathing and facial muscle activation, reducing cortisol and increasing feel-good hormones.

## Nutritional support for nervous system healing

Certain nutrients specifically support nervous system recovery:

- **Omega-3 fatty acids** such as eicosapentaenoic acid (EPA) and docosahexaenoic acid (DHA) reduce neuroinflammation and support membrane health. Aim for 2–3 grams daily of combined EPA and DHA from high-quality fish oil or algae-based supplements.
- **Magnesium** is the 'relaxation mineral', which supports more than 300 enzymatic reactions and helps regulate the stress response. Look for magnesium glycinate, which is easily absorbed and calming.
- **B-complex vitamins** are essential for neurotransmitter production and nervous system function. B vitamins are rapidly depleted during stress, making supplementation often necessary.
- **Adaptogenic herbs** such as ashwagandha, rhodiola and holy basil help modulate the stress response and support adrenal function. These herbs work by supporting the hypothalamic–pituitary–adrenal axis.

### BUILDING YOUR HEALING TOOLKIT

Start small and build gradually:

**Weeks 1–2**

Begin doing breathwork (5 minutes) and one mindfulness practice.

**Weeks 3–4**

Add gentle movement or nature time.

**Weeks 5–6**

Introduce vagus nerve practices.

**Weeks 7–8**

Consider somatic therapy or eye movement desensitisation and reprocessing if trauma is present.

Remember: consistency trumps intensity. The most effective intervention is the one you do regularly. Think of it as compound interest for your nervous system – small, consistent investments yield enormous returns over time.

## THE RIPPLE EFFECT: From survival to thriving

Healing is more than just managing symptoms, it's about shifting from survival mode to a place where your body, mind and emotions function harmoniously. Your body's response to trauma and stress was intelligent; it helped you survive. With understanding and support, you can now help it thrive.

The path forward involves recognising how your past experiences shape your present health and using that knowledge to support recovery. True healing addresses the root of nervous system dysfunction, creating lasting change that ripples through every aspect of your well-being.

Your body may keep score, but it also keeps the capacity for healing. Through these practices, you're not just reducing inflammation but teaching your nervous system that it's safe to rest, restore and thrive.

The journey from surviving to thriving isn't linear – it's more like a spiral staircase where you revisit similar themes at deeper levels. Each time you practise nervous system regulation, you're rewiring your brain for greater resilience and well-being. Your nervous system is remarkably adaptable, and with patience and consistency, it can learn new patterns of safety and ease.

Remember, healing happens in relationship – with yourself, with others and with the natural world. As you develop these practices, you're healing yourself and also contributing to a more regulated, peaceful world for everyone around you.

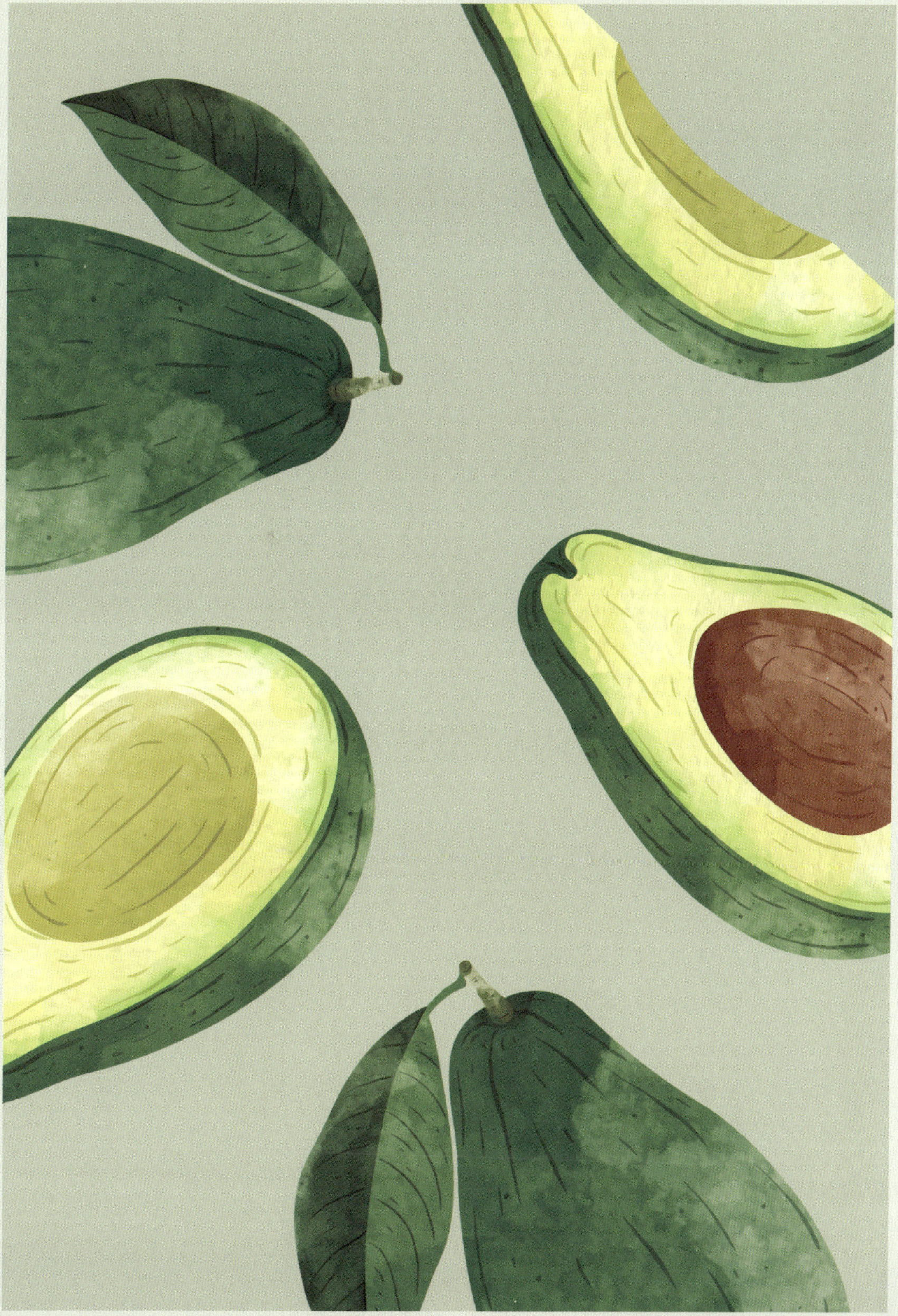

CHAPTER 7

# REWIRE AND RE-BALANCE WITH TRADITIONAL WISDOM AND MODERN TOOLS

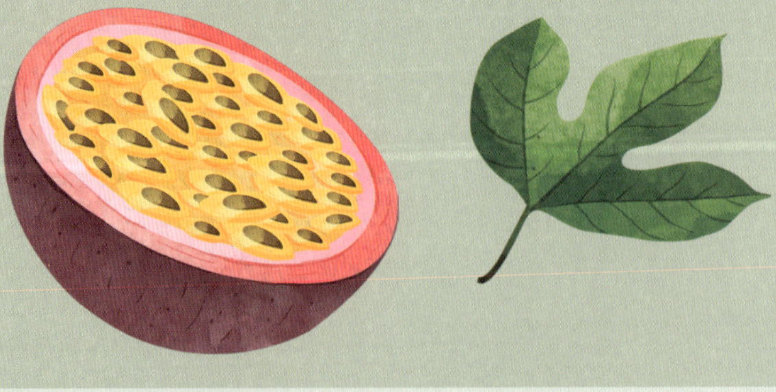

Now that we understand how trauma and chronic stress rewire the nervous system and create inflammatory cascades, let's explore how we can actively restore balance and support your body's natural healing capacity. This involves combining ancient wisdom with modern science to reveal inflammation's roots: at-home practices, strength training and time-tested remedies empower you to reduce inflammation and restore balance.

## WHAT TRADITIONAL MEDICINE TEACHES US ABOUT INFLAMMATION

Long before modern medicine recognised chronic inflammation's dangers, ancient healing traditions like ayurveda and traditional Chinese medicine (TCM) were emphasising body balance to maintain health. These systems view inflammation as disrupted equilibrium, often caused by poor diet, emotional stress or environmental factors. Think of it this way: while Western medicine was busy inventing sophisticated laboratory tests to measure inflammatory markers, traditional healers were already treating the whole person – body, mind and spirit – thousands of years ago.

### AYURVEDA: Know your dosha, know yourself

This holistic system classifies individuals based on their dominant dosha (vata, pitta and kapha), recommending specific anti-inflammatory herbs, foods and lifestyle practices. Ayurveda is like having a personalised user manual for your body.

- **Vata types** (air and space elements) tend towards anxiety and digestive issues when out of balance. They benefit from warming, grounding foods and practices: root vegetables, warm spices and gentle consistent routines.
- **Pitta types** (fire and water elements) are prone to inflammatory conditions when stressed. They require cooling foods and calming practices: cucumber, mint and avoiding excessive heat or intensity.

- **Kapha types** (earth and water elements) may experience sluggish digestion and congestion. They respond well to stimulating, warming interventions: ginger, movement and variety in their routines.

Key Ayurvedic anti-inflammatory allies include the following herbal remedies:

- **Turmeric**, a foundational anti-inflammatory spice
- **Ashwagandha**, an adaptogenic herb for stress management
- **Triphala**, a gentle three-fruit blend supporting digestion and detoxification

## TRADITIONAL CHINESE MEDICINE: HArmonise your qi, harmonise your health

TCM focuses on harmonising qi (life energy) through acupuncture, herbal formulations and dietary therapy. Rather than suppressing inflammation, TCM views it as blocked or misdirected body energy. Forget energy drinks; TCM offers a different approach to boosting vitality through anti-inflammatory herbs such as astragalus (immune-boosting), ginseng (adaptogenic) and reishi mushrooms (calming).

TCM treats inflammation as an imbalance that requires gentle correction rather than aggressive suppression. The beauty of TCM lies in its personalised approach: practitioners assess your individual constitution, lifestyle and current state of health to create a tailored treatment plan. This might include specific herbal formulations, dietary recommendations, acupuncture points and lifestyle modifications designed to restore harmony to your system. By integrating these time-tested insights with contemporary anti-inflammatory strategies, you can take a proactive approach to long-term health that addresses the root causes of inflammation rather than merely managing symptoms.

## THE FOUNDATION: Hydration and gentle cleansing

Before diving into complex interventions, let's address something beautifully simple yet often overlooked: proper hydration. Your body is like a sophisticated water filtration system; when that system becomes sluggish, inflammation accumulates like debris in a blocked drain.

Proper hydration is fundamental to regulating your nervous system. When you're dehydrated, your body struggles to maintain the delicate fluid balance that keeps your cells communicating effectively. The vagus nerve we discussed in Chapter 6 relies on your body having optimal fluid balance to transmit its calming signals effectively. Dehydration creates static in your body's internal communication network. The messages your vagus nerve tries to send about safety and calm become garbled or delayed, making it harder to shift out of sympathetic fight-or-flight mode into the parasympathetic rest-and-digest state that's essential for healing.

Drinking clean, filtered water; electrolyte-enhanced water; or herbal infusions like nettle, dandelion or chamomile tea helps remove inflammatory waste products and keeps the body functioning optimally while supporting your nervous system's capacity for self-regulation (vagal tone).

Simple hydration strategies include the following:

- Start each morning with warm water and lemon to kickstart your lymphatic system and gently stimulate vagal pathways through the throat.
- Aim to drink about 35 ml (1 fl oz) water per kilogram of body weight daily (so if you weigh 64 kg [70 lb], aim for about 2.2 litres [70 fl oz]).
- Add a pinch of high-quality sea salt for natural electrolyte balance that supports nerve conduction.
- Include herbal teas as part of your daily fluid intake: chamomile for evening calm and vagal stimulation, nettle for mineral support, and dandelion for gentle liver support.

Think of proper hydration as giving your internal plumbing system a gentle, daily service while simultaneously supporting your nervous system's ability to regulate inflammation. Love Your Gut powder, which contains diatomaceous earth, provides a gentle cleanse to remove build-up of accumulated waste – like having a professional cleaning service for your digestive tract, but without the hefty bill.

## AT-HOME HEALING: Simple practices for your anti-inflammatory journey

Transform your living room into the ultimate anti-inflammatory laboratory. These simple, science-backed techniques require no prescription and fit into even the busiest schedules. Each method creates measurable biochemical shifts, calming inflammatory pathways and rewiring immune responses.

### LAUGHTER AS MEDICINE: THe best side-effect-free treatment

Even brief moments of genuine laughter (3–5 minutes) increase salivary immunoglobulin A and decrease stress hormones like cortisol. Your body can't tell the difference between real and forced laughter, so even pretending triggers beneficial biochemical changes.

Schedule 5–10 minutes of comedy into your daily routine, create a 'funny folder' on your phone with videos that never fail to make you laugh or try the 'fake it till you make it' approach. Watch funny animal videos, call that friend who always makes you giggle or try laughter yoga (yes, it's a real thing, and yes, it works). Social laughter amplifies the anti-inflammatory benefits even further – sharing funny moments with others creates a compound effect on your immune system.

### COGNITIVE CRAFTING: The meditative power of making

Repetitive, creative activities like knitting, crochet or origami induce a flow state, quieting the brain's rumination centre and increasing anti-inflammatory alpha waves. The key is immersion in the process. There's something deeply satisfying about creating something with your hands while creating calm in your nervous system. Whether you're folding paper cranes or knitting scarves for your community, these activities provide a form of moving meditation that your inflammatory markers like interleukin-6 and CRP will enjoy.

Choose activities that require just enough concentration to keep your mind engaged but not overwhelmed; add complexity as your skills develop. Start with simple projects and focus on the process rather than the outcome (imperfect projects still provide perfect anti-inflammatory benefits). Consider joining online communities or local groups for social connection alongside crafting, which adds another layer of anti-inflammatory benefit through meaningful social interaction.

## JOURNALLING FOR ANTI-INFLAMMATION: Writing your way to wellness

Structured emotional journalling has been shown to reduce pro-inflammatory gene expression in immune cells. This technique lets you release emotional burdens while lowering inflammation. Think of it like creating a dialogue with your immune system and you're writing your way to better health. The act of translating emotions into words helps your brain process and release stored stress, preventing it from manifesting as physical inflammation. Here are some effective techniques:

- **Stream-of-consciousness writing,** where you set a timer for 10 minutes and write whatever comes to mind without editing.
- **Gratitude plus processing,** where you write three things you're grateful for, then explore one challenging emotion or situation.
- **Body-awareness journaling,** where you write about physical sensations, noting areas of tension or discomfort.
- **Future-self letters,** where you write to yourself one year from now, describing your ideal health and how you're working towards it.

The key is consistency rather than perfection – even 5 minutes of honest writing can create measurable shifts in your inflammatory markers.

## STRENGTH TRAINING AND MOBILITY: Building resilience inside and out

Preserving muscle mass through resistance training is essential for your metabolic health, insulin sensitivity and mitochondrial function. Movement and strength-building exercises help stimulate mitophagy, where your ageing mitochondria are replaced with newer, more efficient ones. But here's the thing about strength training and inflammation: it's all about the sweet spot.

The goal is finding that Goldilocks zone – just right for your body's current capacity. Too little movement creates stagnation, allowing inflammatory processes to build up like sediment in a still pond. Too much intense exercise creates excessive inflammatory stress. Consistency wins over intensity; regular, moderate resistance training creates lasting metabolic improvements without triggering excessive inflammatory responses.

### Strength training to cool your inflammatory fires

Compound movements like squats, deadlifts and lunges engage multiple muscle groups simultaneously, maximising metabolic benefits while improving functional strength. These exercises work multiple systems at once while keeping inflammation in check. Start where you are and build consistency and strength progressively.

Bodyweight progressions such as push-ups, pull-ups and dips can be modified for any fitness level and gradually intensified as strength improves. Wall push-ups are just as valuable as floor push-ups when you're starting your journey. Resistance bands provide variable resistance through complete ranges of motion while being gentle on your connective tissues.

Isometric holds such as planks, wall sits and bridges build endurance and stability with minimal joint stress, making them excellent for inflammation-sensitive individuals. These exercises teach your muscles to work efficiently without creating excessive inflammatory by-products. Slow eccentric training, focusing on the lowering phase of movements (like a slow squat), stimulates muscle growth with less overall load, reducing the inflammatory response. It's quality over quantity – slower, more controlled movements may provide better results with less stress.

### JOINT MOBILITY: Keeping your body's hinges well-oiled

Controlled rotations and movements through full ranges of motion for all major joints help maintain the health of your synovial fluid and reduce inflammation build-up. This regular maintenance of your body's moving parts keeps everything flowing smoothly. Spend 5–10 minutes each morning moving through gentle joint rotations: neck, shoulders, hips, ankles. This helps clear overnight stiffness and sets up your body for easier movement throughout the day.

Evening stretches help release tension from the day and promote better sleep quality, which directly impacts your inflammatory markers. Gently stretching before bed creates a transition ritual that signals to your body it's time to shift into repair and recovery mode.

### THE ART OF RECOVERY: When less is more

Aim for 2–3 strength sessions weekly, allowing 48 hours between training the same muscle groups. Listen to your body's inflammation signals: excessive soreness lasting more than 48 hours, disrupted sleep, elevated resting heart rate or persistent fatigue may indicate you're pushing too hard. Recovery is where the magic happens, as your body adapts, strengthens and reduces inflammatory load.

## CREATING YOUR PERSONAL ANTI-INFLAMMATORY TOOLKIT

The beauty of this approach lies in its adaptability. You don't need to implement everything at once – this might create more stress than benefit. Instead, build up gradually, starting with one simple practice and adding others as they become habit. Focus on what feels sustainable and enjoyable, remembering that the most effective anti-inflammatory intervention is the one you'll do consistently.

Consider starting with the foundation: proper hydration and one simple practice like morning water with fulvic humic concentrate combined with 5 minutes of daily laughter. Once this feels natural (usually after a week or two), add gentle movement – perhaps morning joint rotations or evening stretches. As your confidence builds, introduce cognitive practices like journalling or crafting for 10 minutes daily. Finally, begin incorporating strength training twice weekly, starting with bodyweight exercises and progressing as your body adapts.

Remember that setbacks are normal and expected; they're part of the process, not failures. If you miss a day or even a week, simply restart without judgement. The goal isn't perfection; it's progress and consistency over time.

Your body has an incredible capacity for healing and balance. These tools simply help remove the obstacles and create the conditions for your natural healing wisdom to flourish. By integrating traditional wisdom with modern understanding, you're supporting your body's innate ability to heal, balance and thrive.

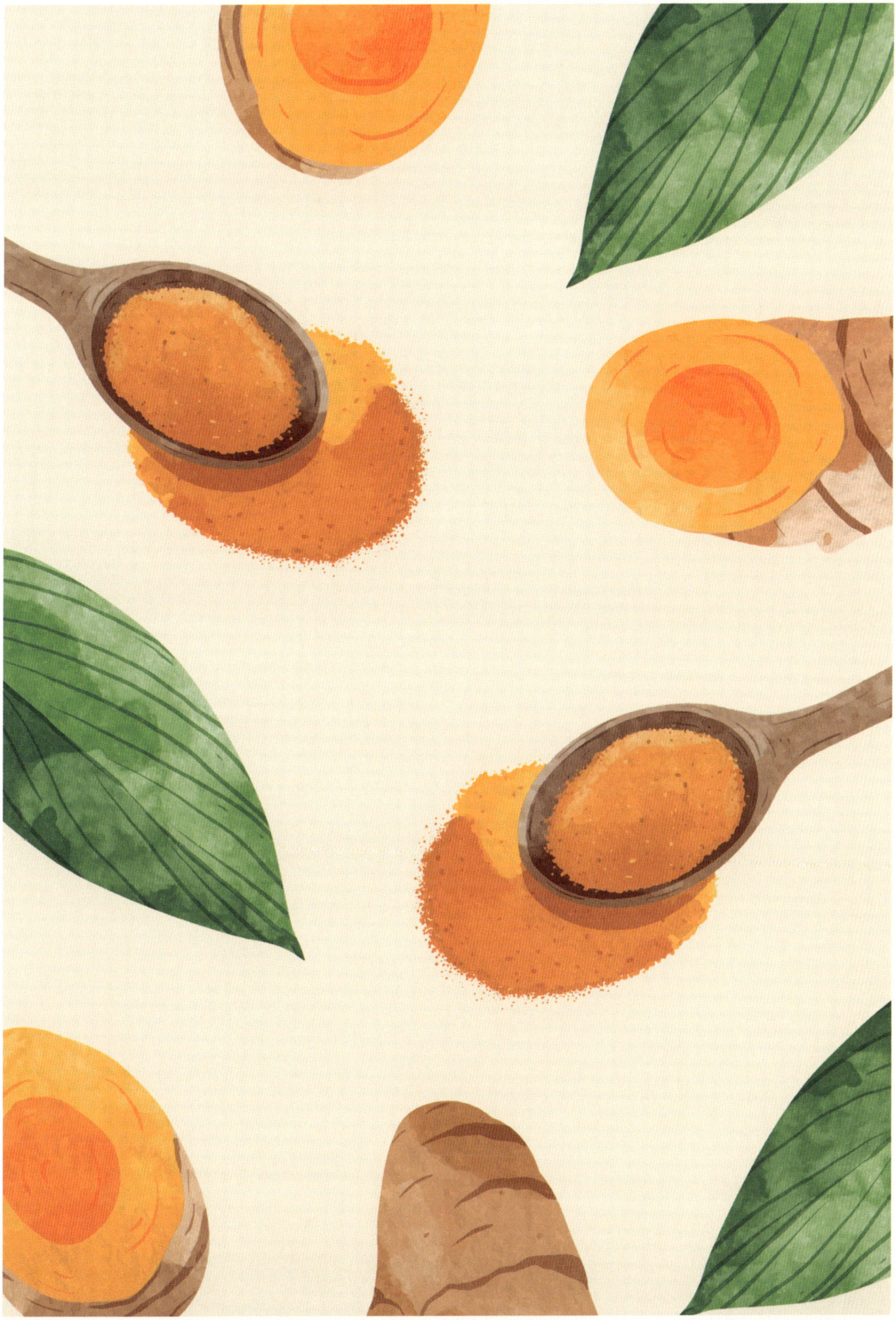

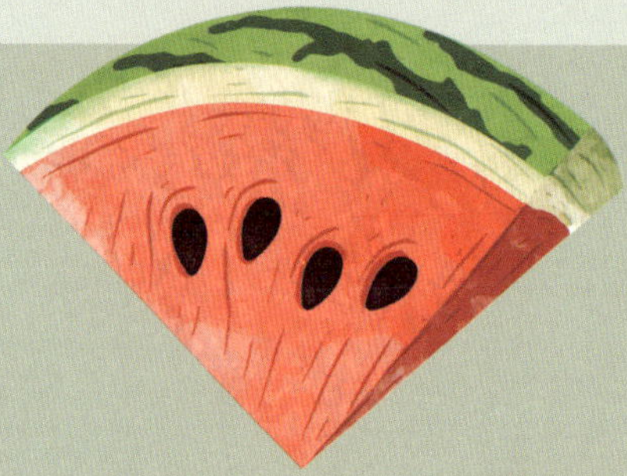

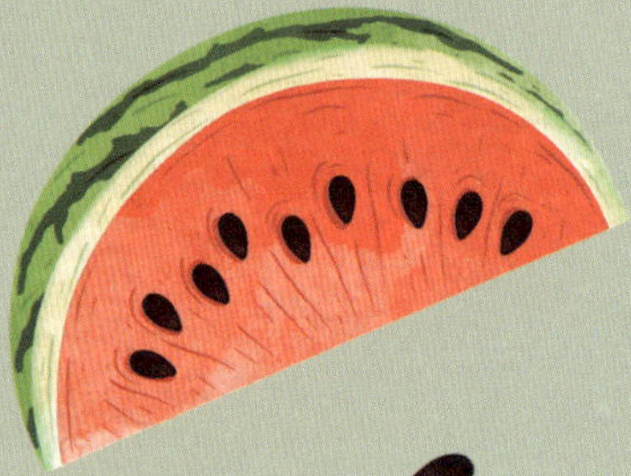

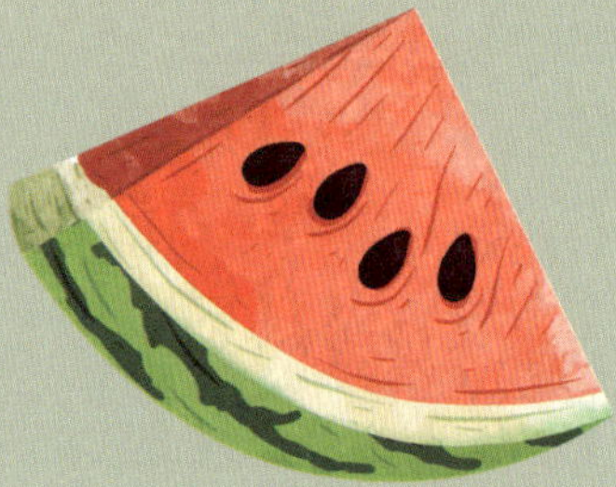

CHAPTER 8

# SUPERCHARGE YOUR CELLS

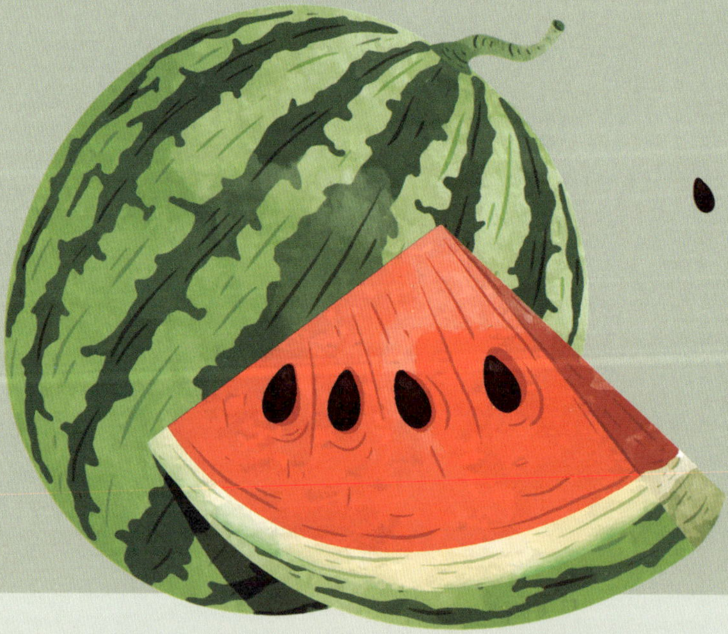

In this chapter, we'll take a tour of the microscopic drama happening inside your body. You'll discover how to evict those troublesome 'zombie cells' – the lazy house guests who won't leave and just sit around causing inflammation. I'll introduce you to your cellular cleaning crew, a process called autophagy. Most importantly, you'll learn how to put this crew to work and supercharge every cell in your body.

## THE CELLULAR SPRING CLEAN YOU NEVER KNEW YOU NEEDED

Imagine if your home had a magical cleaning service that worked around the clock, quietly disposing of broken furniture, clearing out expired items and making space for replacements. That's happening inside your cells every single day through two remarkable processes: autophagy and mitophagy.

Autophagy is like your cellular Marie Kondo – it's constantly asking, 'Does this spark joy for my cell?' If the answer is 'no' (whether it's damaged proteins, worn-out organelles or cellular debris), it gets packaged up and recycled into useful building blocks. Autophagy is essential maintenance that keeps your cells functioning optimally.

Mitophagy takes this cleaning concept to the next level. It's your specialist maintenance crew focused exclusively on your cellular power stations – the mitochondria. When these tiny engines become damaged or inefficient, mitophagy steps in to remove them before they cause trouble, ensuring only the healthiest, most efficient mitochondria remain to fuel your cells.

Here's where it gets exciting: you can actively enhance both these cleaning processes through simple lifestyle choices. You can give your internal cleaning crew better tools, more motivation and optimal working conditions.

## YOUR DAILY CELLULAR SUPERCHARGE ROUTINE

Before we dive into the science, let's start with what you can do today. These simple practices will get your cellular cleaning crew working overtime:

## MORNING CELLULAR ACTIVATION (5–10 MINUTES)

Step outside for natural sunlight exposure, even on cloudy days. This synchronises your cellular clocks and optimises mitochondrial function. Take 10 deep breaths of fresh air to oxygenate your cells, followed by gentle stretching or walking. This morning ritual sets the cellular tone for your entire day.

## MIDDAY CELLULAR MAINTENANCE

Incorporate 20–30 minutes of 'Zone 2' movement – conversational-pace activity where you can still chat but it requires effort. It could be a brisk walk during lunch, cycling to work or steady swimming. This specifically targets mitochondrial efficiency, training your cellular engines to become more powerful and efficient.

## EVENING CELLULAR RECOVERY

Begin your cellular wind-down routine by blocking blue light 2 hours before sleep. Create a cool, dark sleeping environment that supports optimal cellular recovery. After an early dinner at about 6 pm, start your fasting window to allow overnight cellular repair processes to occur – this is when your cleaning crew does their most intensive work.

# YOUR CELLULAR CLEANING ARSENAL:
## The nutrients that do the heavy lifting

Your cellular cleaning team needs specific nutrients to function at their best. Here's your complete cellular nutrition arsenal:

- **Pyrroloquinoline quinone is the cellular construction manager.** This remarkable compound doesn't just support existing mitochondria, it helps create new ones. Pyrroloquinoline quinone (PQQ) oversees the building of fresh, efficient cellular engines. Found naturally in fermented foods and certain vegetables, supplementing with PQQ can significantly boost mitochondrial density, particularly beneficial as we age.
- **Nicotinamide riboside is the energy currency restorer.** As a precursor to NAD+ (nicotinamide adenine dinucleotide), this compound helps maintain your cells' energy currency. NAD+ levels naturally decline with age, dropping by up to 50% between ages 40 and 60. Nicotinamide riboside tops up your cellular bank account, supporting mitochondrial function and cellular repair mechanisms.
- **Magnesium is the unsung cellular hero.** Required for more than 300 enzymatic reactions, magnesium is essential for mitochondrial function. It serves as a cofactor in ATP production – your primary cellular energy currency. Without enough magnesium, your cellular engines can't fire on all cylinders. Magnesium glycinate or malate forms are well-absorbed.
- **B vitamins are the cellular support team.** B vitamins work as a coordinated cleaning crew. B1 helps convert glucose into cellular fuel, B2 is essential for energy production, B3 supports NAD+ production and B5 is crucial for cellular metabolism. Rather than taking them individually, a high-quality B-complex ensures they work together like a well-rehearsed cleaning team.
- **CoQ10 is the cellular protector.** This compound acts like a protective shield for your mitochondria while simultaneously supporting energy

production. CoQ10 levels naturally decline with age, so supplementation is valuable for maintaining cellular energy and protecting against oxidative damage.

These nutrients work better together than in isolation. PQQ builds new mitochondria while CoQ10 optimises their function. Magnesium enhances B-vitamin absorption, and nicotinamide riboside works synergistically with other NAD+ supporting compounds. Taking these supplements with meals improves their absorption, particularly for fat-soluble compounds like CoQ10.

## THE SPECIALIST TECHNICIANS: Advanced mitochondrial support

Beyond the core team, certain nutrients act like specialist technicians for your mitochondria. These nutrients are your cellular pit crew – each member has a specific job, but together they create a high-performance team:

- **Creatine** acts as a cellular energy buffer, storing and quickly releasing energy when your mitochondria need extra support. It's beneficial for brain function and physical performance. Use high-purity forms (creatine monohydrate) and ensure it's free from impurities and additives.
- **Carnitine** helps transport fatty acids into mitochondria for energy production, like a dedicated fuel delivery service for your cellular engines. Carnitine can interact with blood thinners and certain medications, so check with your health professional before using.
- **Fulvic humic concentrate** enhances cellular nutrient absorption and supports mitochondrial function while providing trace minerals that act as cellular cofactors.
- **Berberine** supports mitochondrial biogenesis and helps optimise cellular energy metabolism; it's beneficial for metabolic health. Some people experience mild gastrointestinal symptoms, so always check with your health professional and avoid when pregnant or breastfeeding.
- **Resveratrol** activates longevity pathways and supports mitochondrial function, helping your cellular engines age more gracefully.

| SCOPE | TARGETS | PURPOSE | HOW TO SUPERCHARGE IT |
|---|---|---|---|
| General cellular clean-up and recycling | Various cellular components (proteins, lipids, organelles) | Maintain cellular health, respond to stress | Kilojoule restriction, intermittent fasting, exercise, adequate sleep, stress management |
| Selective removal of damaged mitochondria | Specifically targets mitochondria | Maintain mitochondrial health, prevent inflammation | Mitochondrial-specific nutrients such as PQQ, creatine, carnitine, fulvic humic concentrate and CoQ10 supplementation |

## Movement that supercharges your cells

Your cellular cleaning crew responds beautifully to the right kind of movement. Here's how to get them working at peak efficiency:

- **Zone 2 cardio** is the cellular sweet spot. This is your mitochondrial training ground. During Zone 2 cardio, your mitochondria become more efficient at using oxygen and fat for fuel. Aim for 30–45 minutes of brisk walking, easy cycling or steady swimming.
- **Lymphatic drainage** is your cellular waste collection. Your lymphatic system is like your body's rubbish collection service, but it doesn't have a central pump – it relies on movement. Gentle rebounding (bouncing on a mini-trampoline), dry brushing or walking helps move cellular waste products out of tissues. This prevents accumulated waste from interfering with cellular function.
- **Vibration therapy** is a gentle cellular massage. Whole-body vibration platforms create mechanical stress that encourages cellular adaptation and improved circulation. Even 10–15 minutes can provide benefits without exhausting you. It's useful if you have mobility limitations or to complement other movement.

## CELLULAR HYDRATION: The foundation of efficient cleaning

Proper cellular hydration goes far beyond drinking eight glasses of water daily. Your cellular cleaning crew needs the right fluid environment to function effectively:

- **Electrolyte balance is the cellular communication network.** Sodium, potassium, magnesium and calcium create electrical gradients across cell membranes that your cells need to communicate. Adding a pinch of high-quality sea salt to water or using fulvic humic concentrate can improve cellular hydration more effectively than water alone.
- **Spring water – what cells prefer.** Some research suggests that water found naturally in springs may be better utilised by cells. Try drinking natural spring water, using certain filtration systems or storing water in glass containers for additional cellular benefits.

## TIMING YOUR CELLULAR RECOVERY: The circadian connection

Your cellular cleaning crew works on a schedule, just like any professional cleaning service. Understanding this timing can dramatically improve their efficiency.

- **Light exposure is your cellular timekeeper.** Morning sunlight doesn't just help you feel awake – it actively optimises mitochondrial function by signalling your cells to ramp up energy production. Even 10–15 minutes of morning light exposure can significantly impact your cellular function throughout the day.
- **Manage evening light to protect the night shift.** Just as morning light energises your cellular team, evening blue light exposure disrupts their natural recovery cycles. Blue-light-blocking glasses or reducing screen time for 2 hours before bed supports your cells' night-shift cleaning and repair processes.

- **Quality sleep is when the deep cleaning happens.** During deep sleep, your cells shift into intensive repair mode. This is when autophagy and mitophagy work most efficiently, clearing out damaged components and preparing your mitochondria for the next day's demands. When you sleep poorly, your cellular cleaning crew can't complete their essential maintenance routines.

## EVICTING THE ZOMBIE CELLS: Natural senolytic strategies

Now, let's talk about those problematic zombie cells – senescent cells that hang around like unwanted house guests, causing inflammation and making your tissues dysfunctional. The good news? Nature provides excellent eviction notices.

Inflammaging (the combination of inflammation and ageing) describes the low-grade, chronic inflammation that gradually increases as we age. This persistent inflammatory background noise drives most age-related diseases and creates a hostile environment for your healthy cells.

### NATURE'S EVICTION SQUAD: Natural senolytics

Several plant compounds act as natural senolytic agents, helping to clear these cellular troublemakers:

- **Fisetin** is found in strawberries, apples and onions. It selectively eliminates senescent cells and reduces inflammation. Time to stock up on strawberries!
- **Quercetin** is present in capers, apples, onions and berries. It is both an antioxidant and senolytic, especially when combined with other compounds.
- **Curcumin** is the active compound in turmeric, which helps reduce inflammatory signalling from senescent cells and supports cellular repair mechanisms.

- **Resveratrol** is found in grapes and blueberries. It has longevity-promoting effects by activating sirtuins, which help counteract cellular ageing.
- **EGCG** is a key antioxidant in green tea, which helps reduce inflammation from ageing cells – a delicious way to sip your way to cellular health.

## YOUR COMPLETE CELLULAR SUPPORT STRATEGY

### CELLULAR FRIENDS (welcome these daily)

- Morning sunlight and natural light cycles
- Nutrient-dense, colourful foods
- Regular Zone 2 movement
- Quality sleep in a cool, dark room
- Intermittent fasting periods
- Clean air and filtered water
- Stress management and relaxation
- Gentle heat and cold therapy
- Natural, non-toxic products
- Social connections and laughter

### CELLULAR ENEMIES (show these the door)

- Artificial light after sunset
- Processed foods and excess sugar
- Sedentary lifestyle and chronic stress
- Poor sleep quality and irregular schedules
- Constant eating without fasting breaks
- Environmental toxins and pollutants
- Chronic inflammation and oxidative stress
- Chemical-laden products and excessive electromagnetic field exposure
- Social isolation and chronic negativity

## YOUR NEXT STEPS: Putting it all together

The journey to optimal cellular health is like creating the perfect cleaning routine for your home – it requires consistency, the right tools and patience to see results. Here's how to start:

- **This week,** begin your daily cellular routine – morning sunlight, Zone 2 movement and evening light management.
- **This month,** add key nutrients like magnesium, B-complex and CoQ10 to support your cellular cleaning crew.
- **This quarter,** incorporate natural senolytic foods (berries, green tea, turmeric) and gentle intermittent fasting.
- **This year,** create a sustainable rhythm that includes quality sleep, stress management and regular movement.

Remember, your cells are constantly working behind the scenes to keep you thriving. By supporting autophagy and mitophagy, providing premium fuel through targeted nutrition and creating optimal conditions through proper timing and lifestyle choices, you're investing in decades of vitality ahead. Your cellular cleaning crew is ready to work; now you have the blueprint to help them excel.

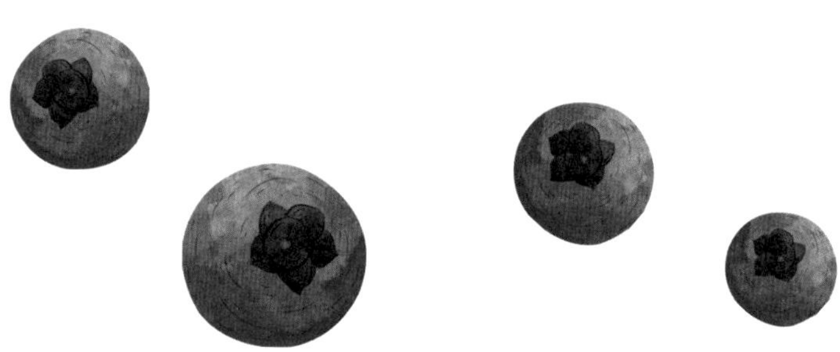

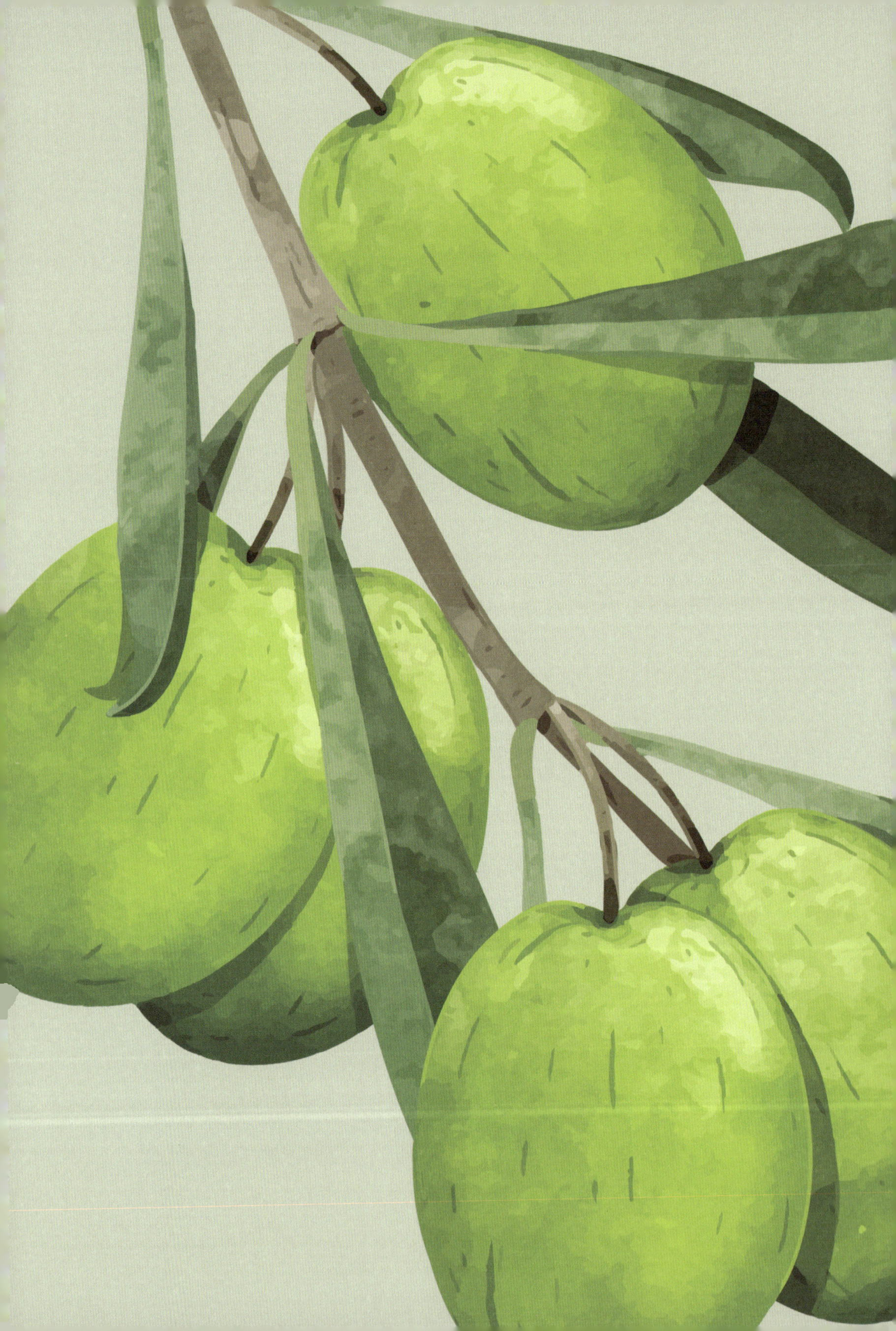

PART 3

# YOUR PERSONAL MAP PROTOCOL

This is where transformation happens. Using everything we've learned about inflammation and nervous system regulation, I've designed a protocol that reduces inflammation, calms your nervous system and supercharges every cell. My comprehensive Mediterranean Anti-inflammatory Plan (MAP) is designed to reduce inflammation and restore your health. The chapters ahead provide you with practical tools, including targeted nutrition, meal planning and 60 delicious Mediterranean-style recipes, for you to implement the MAP protocol.

CHAPTER 9

# YOUR PERSONALISED INFLAMMATION SELF-ASSESSMENT

An anti-inflammatory lifestyle is your ticket to a longer, brighter and more supercharged future. Chronic inflammation underpins nearly every significant age-related ailment, from dodgy hearts to foggy brains and creaky joints.

This chapter is your friendly compass for feeling better and building a body that stands the test of time – a pension plan for your cells. By marrying the sage advice from traditional medicine with our modern scientific toolkit, you can craft a sustainable inflammation-taming lifestyle that adds quality years to your life. And let's be honest – what good is reaching 90 if you can't remember where you put your birthday cake or don't have enough energy to blow out the candles?

## WHAT'S YOUR FIRE RATING?

Inflammation doesn't just lurk in the shadows – it announces itself in various ways throughout your body and mind. Physically, inflammation can manifest as persistent fatigue that no amount of sleep seems to fix, mysterious aches and pains that migrate around your body, digestive dramas that disrupt your daily routine and (if ignored long enough) chronic illnesses that require medical intervention.

The effects don't stop there. Mentally, inflammation can wrap your brain in cotton wool, creating that frustrating sense of fogginess, making concentration feel monumental and gradually dimming your cognitive sparkle.

Even your emotional landscape bears inflammation's sticky fingerprints. It can amplify your stress response, trigger anxiety spirals, send your mood on a roller-coaster ride and deepen feelings of depression. But the underlying cause isn't just 'life'; it's actual biochemical changes in your body.

Now we know how to identify the signs and symptoms of inflammation, let's look at what can be quantified.

The following quiz will help you personally assess your current inflammation levels by identifying common signs and symptoms. Reflect honestly on each question, considering your experiences over the past month to gain insights into your body's inflammatory state and what steps you might take towards better health.

If you're worried, please consult your healthcare provider for personalised advice and to discuss relevant inflammatory markers like CRP, ESR, interleukin-6 and D-dimer. When combined with your self-assessment, the results of these tests can provide a more complete picture of your inflammatory status.

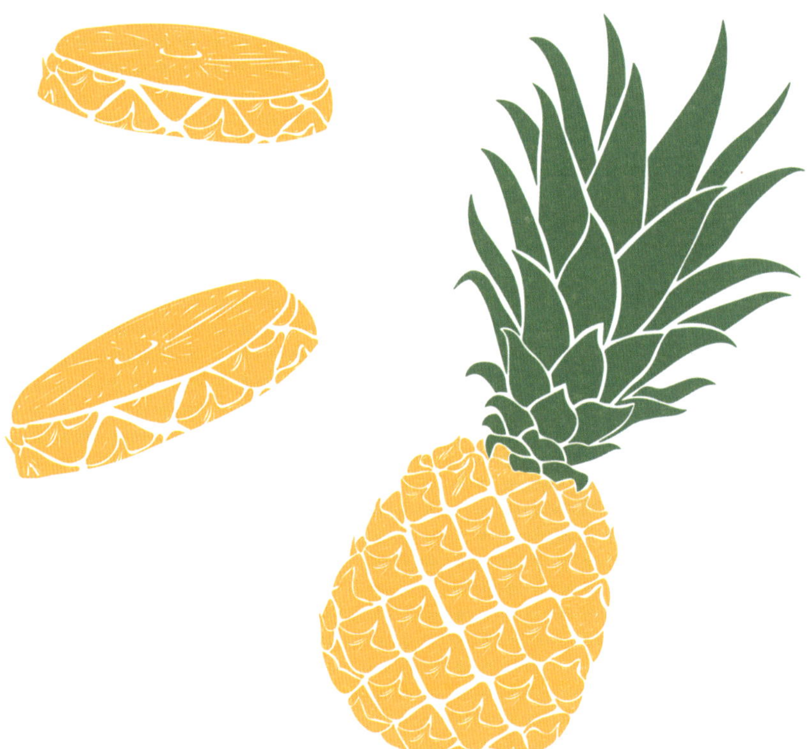

# QUIZ – YOUR CURRENT INFLAMMATION LEVELS

Score each statement that follows based on how frequently you've experienced these symptoms or conditions over the past 4 weeks using the following options:

**0 – Never | 1 – Rarely | 2 – Occasionally | 3 – Frequently | 4 – Almost always**

1. **I experience persistent fatigue or low energy levels.**
2. **I often have joint pain, stiffness or swelling.**
3. **My digestion frequently feels uncomfortable (bloating, gas, diarrhoea, constipation).**
4. **I regularly have headaches or migraines.**
5. **I notice my mood fluctuates, including increased anxiety or depressive feelings.**
6. **I experience skin irritations, such as eczema, psoriasis, acne or unexplained rashes.**
7. **My sleep quality is poor or disrupted regularly.**
8. **I have allergies or sensitivities to foods or environmental triggers.**
9. **I feel mentally foggy or have trouble concentrating.**
10. **My muscles often ache or feel sore without significant physical exertion.**
11. **I gain weight easily or struggle to lose weight despite healthy efforts.**
12. **I frequently feel physically unwell or like I'm coming down with something.**
13. **My stress levels are consistently high or difficult to manage.**
14. **I engage in physical activity fewer than three times per week.**
15. **I have a medical history of autoimmune conditions, chronic illness or inflammatory diseases.**
16. **I've previously had elevated inflammatory markers, such as ESR or CRP, in blood tests.**

## SCORING

### 0–12 POINTS

Low inflammation. Your inflammation levels appear minimal. Maintain your current healthy lifestyle and enjoy my delicious recipes.

### 13–28 POINTS

Moderate inflammation. Some inflammation is present. Consider reviewing your diet and lifestyle for factors that may contribute.

### 29–44 POINTS

High inflammation. Significant inflammation is likely present. Focus on consuming anti-inflammatory foods, reducing stress and improving sleep, and consider seeking professional advice.

### 45–64 POINTS

Severe inflammation. High levels of inflammation are probable. Making immediate lifestyle adjustments and seeking professional evaluation are strongly recommended.

# WHAT YOUR SCORE MEANS AND NEXT STEPS

What were your quiz results? If you scored high on question 3, which assesses digestive discomfort, it may indicate inflammation triggered by food sensitivities. Try keeping a detailed food diary to track your meals and correlating symptoms. This can help you identify potential triggers you may not be aware of.

Regardless of your score, making lifestyle changes can significantly reduce your inflammation and improve overall health. Biologically, incorporating anti-inflammatory foods, engaging in regular physical activity, practising stress-reduction techniques and prioritising quality sleep can help decrease your body's production of pro-inflammatory cytokines, regulate immune responses and support a balanced gut microbiome.

Consider making gradual changes to your diet (for more, see the next chapter), physical activity routine, stress management and sleep habits, and monitor them over time. Check in with yourself weekly and monthly to see how you are progressing. If your score suggests significant inflammation, seek professional guidance from a healthcare provider or clinical nutritionist so they can tailor a specific plan to your needs.

CHAPTER 10

# TARGETED NUTRITION AND SUPPLEMENTATION TO REDUCE INFLAMMATION

I have some brilliant news! Your kitchen cupboard is brimming with anti-inflammatory allies just waiting to be recruited. This chapter isn't about bland, restrictive eating or swallowing handfuls of supplements. Instead I'll guide you through the fascinating world of targeted nutrition – from the mighty polyphenols in your morning berries to the gut-healing magic of calming foods.

My personalised 'eat to heal' protocol, known as MAP, uses targeted nutrition with superfoods, phytonutrients and strategic supplementation to combat chronic inflammation and support healing. We'll explore how specific nutrients can switch off inflammatory pathways; why your gut bacteria are your inflammation-fighting partners; and how plant-based compounds, micronutrients and adaptogens enhance immune resilience – approaches I've successfully used in my clinic for years.

To effectively support your body against inflammation, you need a comprehensive plan that focuses on taking in essential nutrients, optimising gut health, reducing systemic inflammation and supporting the mitochondria (your body's cellular engines). You can use the anti-inflammatory nutritional strategies independently or integrate them into your existing healthcare plan. They are designed to enhance energy levels, support natural healing processes and address the root causes of inflammation while creating a personalised strategy that actually fits into your real life.

## TRIPLE THREAT PROTOCOL

**• Inflammation • Stress • Energy**

One protocol, three powerful results. By combining anti-inflammatory nutrition, stress-reduction techniques and targeted supplements, you'll lower inflammation, soothe your nervous system and ignite cellular energy.

## YOUR TAILOR-MADE ANTI-INFLAMMATORY PLAN

Bio-individuality matters tremendously when addressing inflammation. Testing inflammatory markers like CRP, ESR and cytokines can help tailor interventions to your specific needs. If you'd like to look further into your symptoms, consider taking the following tests:

- **Genetic** testing to identify predispositions to inflammatory conditions
- **Gut microbiome** analysis such as gastrointestinal mapping to assess bacterial balance and diversity
- **Food sensitivity** testing to identify personal inflammatory triggers
- **Nutrient status** assessment to identify deficiencies requiring attention

Everyone's biochemistry varies so use this chapter as a guide and consult with your healthcare provider to ensure you're making the right choices for your situation.

## BUILDING THE BASE: The key ingredients to inflammation-free living

The cornerstone of inflammation control begins with phytonutrient-rich, micronutrient-dense foods that actively modulate your immune pathways. These compounds work at a cellular level to combat oxidative stress, regulate inflammatory cytokines (signalling proteins) and support your cells' energy production.

*I worked with a patient, Bella, who was suffering from debilitating joint pain and fatigue. She had tried multiple medications with little success. When she transitioned to an anti-inflammatory diet rich in omega-3s, polyphenols and gut-healing foods, the change was remarkable. Within 3 months, she reported improved energy levels, reduced pain and better digestion. It was a testament to the power of strategic nutrition.*

## GUT FIRST: The secret to a calm and healthy body

Complementing the traditional approaches and mind–body practices we've already covered, targeted nutritional support provides the biochemical foundation for controlling inflammation.

If you're experiencing gut issues such as bloating, motility problems, gas, pain or tiredness after eating, you need to address your gut health before proceeding with other interventions. My comprehensive 'Four step gut-healing reset' (see Chapter 5) will help you reset your digestive system. Once you've completed the reset, return to this chapter for the next step.

## SUPERCHARGE WITH PHYTONUTRIENTS, YOUR BODY'S NATURAL ANTI-INFLAMMATORY WEAPONS

Phytonutrients are bioactive compounds found in plants that regulate inflammation by modulating key pathways like nuclear factor kappa B (NF-κB) and cyclooxygenase-2 (COX-2), which are central players in chronic inflammatory processes.

When I learned about the power of polyphenols, I started incorporating more berries, green tea and dark chocolate into my own diet. The difference? Fewer headaches, better digestion and improved mental clarity.

Key phytonutrients to include in your diet:

- **Polyphenol-rich foods** like berries, green tea, dark chocolate and extra virgin olive oil help regulate inflammatory gene expression.
- **Carotenoids** found in brightly coloured fruits and vegetables such as pumpkin, sweet potatoes and carrots are potent antioxidants.
- **Flavonoids** in citrus fruits, onions, and green and black tea reduce inflammatory mediators like TNF and interleukin-6.

- **Sulforaphane** is a remarkable compound found in broccoli sprouts and other cruciferous vegetables. It enhances detoxification and cellular defence mechanisms against oxidative stress.

## BALANCING YOUR PLATE AND HOW TO MASTER MACRONUTRIENTS FOR INFLAMMATION CONTROL

Beyond individual nutrients, how we balance macronutrients in our daily diet plays a critical role in inflammation management. In my clinic, patients benefit from having a strategic balance of proteins, fats and carbohydrates to maintain metabolic stability.

**Protein** found in amino acids like glycine (from collagen and bone broth) and glutamine help repair the gut lining, reducing inflammation-driven intestinal permeability.

**Fats** that include a favourable omega-3 to omega-6 ratio are key to downregulating pro-inflammatory eicosanoids. Prioritising fatty fish (such as wild-caught salmon, mackerel and trout), linseeds (flaxseeds) and extra virgin olive oil over processed seed oils can significantly reduce inflammatory burden.

**Carbohydrates** can contribute to insulin resistance and inflammation. Instead of a diet high in refined sugars, opt for fibre-rich, low-glycaemic index carbohydrates (such as legumes, quinoa and root vegetables) to help stabilise blood glucose levels and promote gut health.

Food-combining principles offer suggestions on pairing these macronutrients and their significant impact on your digestion and inflammation levels. Some patients have reported improved symptoms when they strategically combine protein with healthy fats for optimal satiety and gut repair. This approach may work by promoting blood glucose stability and reducing inflammatory food combinations that can trigger digestive distress.

## NATURAL SUPERCHARGERS: The inflammation fighters you didn't know you needed

Beyond the foundational macronutrient strategies, some remarkable compounds can significantly amplify our anti-inflammatory efforts.

### Curcumin, the queen of compounds

Building on the traditional wisdom discussed in Chapter 7, modern research confirms that curcumin, the active compound in turmeric can block NF-κB, reduce COX-2 activity and inhibit pro-inflammatory cytokines like TNF. Studies suggest that curcumin supplementation can be as effective as NSAIDs (like ibuprofen) for managing inflammatory conditions such as arthritis and inflammatory bowel disease.

To use, pair turmeric with black pepper (which contains piperine) and healthy fats to enhance bioavailability. My Love Your Gut, Super Potent Curcumin provides a highly concentrated and bioavailable form of curcumin for therapeutic use (for more on nutrients and supplements, see Appendix 3).

### Omega-3s, the fatty anti-inflammation heroes

Found in fatty fish, omega-3 fatty acids (EPA and DHA) can help reduce inflammation, and are beneficial for joint health, cognitive function and cardiovascular inflammation. Good sources of omega-3s include wild-caught salmon, mackerel, linseeds (flaxseeds), walnuts and algae-based omega-3 supplements.

### Ginger and garlic, the dynamic duo of natural COX-2 inhibitors

Ginger contains gingerols and shogaols, which can help inhibit inflammatory enzymes similar to pharmaceutical anti-inflammatories. Garlic is rich in allicin, a compound that enhances immune modulation and reduces oxidative stress. To use, add freshly grated ginger to herbal teas and incorporate raw garlic in dressings or fermented preparations.

# GUT HEALTH = INFLAMMATION CONTROL

## The gut inflammation connection

Recent research has highlighted the role of gut microbiota in regulating inflammation throughout the body. Researchers isolated five strains of helpful gut bacteria, which could lead to new treatments for inflammatory bowel disease and potentially help prevent some forms of bowel cancer. Commensal gut bacteria have been found to induce the production of T cells (a type of white blood cell) that help maintain gut health by counteracting inflammation.

Emerging research is identifying specific strains of probiotics that may have potent anti-inflammatory effects. Strains like *Lactobacillus rhamnosus* GG and *Bifidobacterium infantis* 35624 have demonstrated particular benefits for inflammatory conditions.

## Love Your Gut Synbiotic for gut health and immune function

This is a comprehensive formula designed to optimise gut health and immune function. It contains prebiotics, probiotics and dietary fibre, along with a five-strain probiotic blend featuring *L. acidophilus*, *B. bifidum*, *B. longum*, *B. lactis* and *L. brevis*. These strains work synergistically to support digestive health and reduce inflammation. *L. acidophilus* has potent anti-inflammatory effects, reducing pro-inflammatory cytokines and markers like NF-κB and COX-2.

*Bifidobacterium* strains have been shown to reduce respiratory infection symptoms and promote immune health. These strains work together to decrease pro-inflammatory interleukin-8 and enhance secretion of anti-inflammatory interleukin-10. The probiotic strains in Love Your Gut Synbiotic improve the composition of your gut microbiome, enhance your intestinal barrier, regulate cytokine production and produce beneficial metabolites like short-chain fatty acids. I formulated this comprehensive formula to support your gut and immune function.

## YOUR GUT-BRAIN-CELL CONNECTION: The healing triangle

Everything is connected. A healthy gut supports a balanced brain and energised cells. Probiotics, fibre-rich foods and mindful eating create a healing loop – reducing inflammation, calming the mind and fuelling every cell with what it needs to thrive.

Feed your gut–brain connection to address your mood and inflammation. Cutting-edge trials have identified specific bacterial strains (*L. plantarum* PS128 and *B. longum* 1714) that directly modulate the vagus nerve and reduce plasma kynurenine levels (a metabolite linked to depression and systemic inflammation). These 'mind-altering' microbes create a beneficial feedback loop among your gut, brain and immune system.

## Gut health, prebiotics and detoxification support

**Fulvic humic concentrate** is a unique formula that aids mineral absorption, detoxification and your cells' energy production. It is also a powerful prebiotic (food for beneficial bacteria in the gut), promoting a healthy gut microbiome by enhancing the growth of beneficial bacterial. It supports gut barrier integrity, making it beneficial for leaky gut by improving nutrient absorption and reducing inflammation.

**Diatomaceous earth** is a natural food-grade ingredient that helps cleanse the digestive system, supporting microbiome balance and reducing gut-derived inflammation.

**Apple cider vinegar** capsules can support digestion, improve insulin sensitivity and help regulate inflammatory pathways.

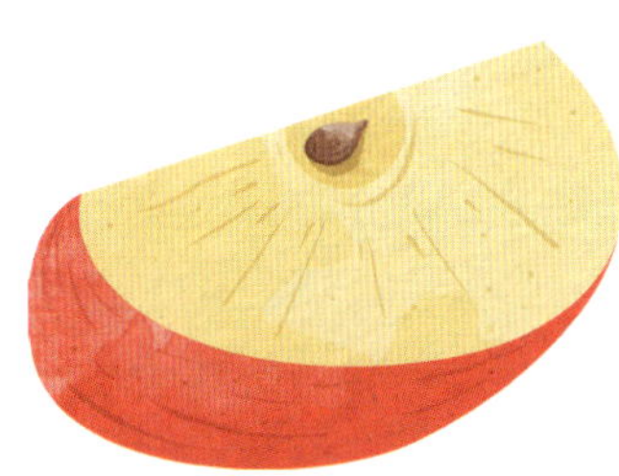

## BUTYRATE, THE GUT'S SECRET WEAPON AGAINST INFLAMMATION

One of the most exciting developments in understanding gut-related inflammation is the role of short-chain fatty acids, particularly butyrate. Beneficial gut bacteria produce these compounds when they ferment dietary fibre and resistant starch.

Butyrate is the primary energy source for colonocytes (colon cells) and helps maintain gut barrier integrity. Recent studies show that butyrate:

- **reduces intestinal permeability** by strengthening tight junctions between cells
- **activates anti-inflammatory pathways** via histone deacetylase inhibition
- **regulates T-regulatory cells**, which help control immune responses
- **maintains colonic oxygen balance**, favouring beneficial bacteria.

Increase your consumption of prebiotic fibre, which is found in foods like Jerusalem artichokes, chicory root, dandelion greens, leeks, onions and garlic. Prebiotics feed the beneficial bacteria that produce butyrate and other short-chain fatty acids. Resistant starch, found in cooked then cooled potatoes, green bananas and legumes, is another excellent butyrate precursor.

## ANTIOXIDANTS AND ADAPTOGENS, THE ULTIMATE TAG TEAM

A diet rich in antioxidants and adaptogens reduces inflammation by combating oxidative stress, supporting gut health and enhancing immune function.

- **Love Your Gut, Golden Gut Blend** is a powerful combination of anti-inflammatory spices, including turmeric, cinnamon and ginger, designed to support gut and immune health. I love adding it to my morning smoothies, golden lattes or even sprinkling it over roasted vegetables for an extra anti-inflammatory boost.

- **Collagen,** an essential protein in the body, supports your joint health, your gut lining integrity and skin elasticity, while reducing inflammation. I mix collagen into my morning coffee, blend it into nourishing soups or whip it into smoothies to keep my skin glowing and my gut happy.
- **Targeted nutritional support** can help to further enhance your gut health and combat inflammation. Certain nutrients and compounds work synergistically to repair the gut lining, regulate stress responses and improve your cells' energy production, all of which are essential for your overall well-being.

## NEXT LEVEL HEALING: Advanced strategies to tame chronic inflammation

### SPMs, the cutting-edge approach to fighting inflammation naturally

The latest inflammation research is shifting from simply suppressing inflammation to actively resolving it. Specialised pro-resolving mediators (SPMs) represent this cutting-edge approach. These lipid compounds (including resolvins, protectins and maresins) are derived from omega-3 fatty acids and actively trigger the resolution phase of inflammation.

Unlike traditional anti-inflammatories that merely block inflammatory pathways, SPMs:

- promote clearance of inflammatory debris
- support tissue regeneration
- reduce pain signals
- return tissue to homeostasis.

SPMs are available as supplements, but you can increase your body's production by consuming ample omega-3 fatty acids from sources like wild-caught fatty fish or algae-based supplements.

## ACTIVATE YOUR NRF2 PATHWAY: A natural way to fight inflammation

The Nrf2 (Nuclear factor erythroid 2-related factor 2) pathway is often called the master regulator of antioxidant defences. When activated, it triggers the production of numerous protective enzymes that combat oxidative stress and inflammation in the cells.

As well as sulforaphane from broccoli sprouts, Nrf2 activators include:

- pterostilbene found in blueberries
- triterpenoids from olives and olive oil
- rosemary extract (carnosic acid)
- curcumin, which works partially through Nrf2 activation.

These compounds help reduce oxidative stress and inflammation by enhancing the body's own antioxidant systems rather than providing antioxidants directly.

## Enzyme therapy and targeted approaches

Proteolytic enzymes are gaining renewed attention for their systemic anti-inflammatory effects. Unlike digestive enzymes, which work primarily in the gut, proteolytic enzymes taken between meals enter the bloodstream to help break down inflammatory proteins and immune complexes throughout the body.

Key proteolytic enzymes with anti-inflammatory properties include:

- bromelain from pineapple
- papain from papaya
- nattokinase from fermented soybeans
- serrapeptase originally isolated from silkworms.

These enzymes can help reduce swelling, pain and fibrin deposits that contribute to inflammatory conditions. They're particularly helpful for recovery from exercise-induced inflammation, joint discomfort and respiratory inflammation.

### Inflammation tests

The field of personalised inflammation testing has evolved significantly in recent years. Beyond standard CRP and ESR tests, consider these newer, more comprehensive assessments:

- **GlycA** (glycoprotein acetylation) is a novel nuclear magnetic resonance marker that measures glycosylated proteins, providing a stable assessment of systemic inflammation with fewer fluctuations than CRP.
- **Cytokine panels** measure specific inflammatory mediators like interleukin-6, TNF and interleukin-1 beta to identify potentially overactive inflammatory pathways.
- **Oxidised LDL** measures cholesterol particles damaged by oxidative stress, which trigger inflammatory responses in blood vessels.
- **Advanced gut permeability** tests assess the integrity of the intestinal barrier, a crucial factor in systemic inflammation.

These tests help create a more tailored approach to managing inflammation by identifying your unique inflammatory patterns and triggers.

## SUPPLEMENT YOUR HEALING WITH TARGETED SUPPORT

While diet is your anti-inflammation foundation, certain supplements provide extra benefits. The following compounds have been extensively studied for their effects on inflammatory pathways and immune function.

Nutritional allies to support your anti-inflammatory goals:

- L-glutamine helps repair the gut barrier and reduces permeability.
- Adaptogens, such as ashwagandha and rhodiola, help modulate the hypothalamic–pituitary–adrenal axis and mitigate stress-related gut dysfunction.

- Magnesium aids in relaxing the nervous system and supports digestion by reducing gut spasms.
- Nutrients like PQQ, creatine, carnitine and CoQ10 enhance the cells' energy production, which is often compromised in chronic inflammation.

## **SUPPLEMENT SMARTS: How to choose and use supplements effectively**

Not all supplements are necessary for everyone because individual needs vary based on lab results, symptoms and inflammatory markers. Important considerations when supplementing:

- Certain compounds, such as curcumin, resveratrol and vitamin D, require fat for absorption.
- Iron benefits from pairing with vitamin C to enhance absorption.
- Excessive supplementation can cause nutrient imbalances – too much omega-3 can lead to blood thinning, while an overabundance of zinc may deplete copper levels.

A well-balanced approach ensures that supplements support, rather than disrupt, overall health. Always consult with a qualified healthcare practitioner before beginning any supplement regimen.

## Strategic control, a blueprint for tackling inflammation naturally

Integrating targeted nutrition, strategic supplementation and anti-inflammatory compounds into your daily routine gives you a personalised, science-driven approach to inflammation regulation. The small, intentional choices can create long-term health resilience, enhance cognitive function and promote longevity.

Chronic inflammation demands a comprehensive approach, which involves:

- identifying your needs through appropriate testing
- leveraging the power of polyphenols and antioxidants from whole foods
- maintaining a balanced intake of macronutrients
- incorporating natural anti-inflammatory agents like curcumin
- ensuring you consume enough omega-3 fatty acids
- eating ginger and garlic, natural COX-2 inhibitors
- supporting your gut health through detoxification, probiotics and adaptogens.

And remember, it's not about perfection but consistency. One anti-inflammatory meal at a time, one lifestyle tweak at a time and before you know it, you're not just surviving – you're thriving.

Start small: swap refined oils for olive oil, add a turmeric latte to your morning routine or eat more omega-3-rich foods. Every step counts on your journey towards reduced inflammation and vibrant health.

For the full table of nutrients, supplements and peptides, see Appendix 3.

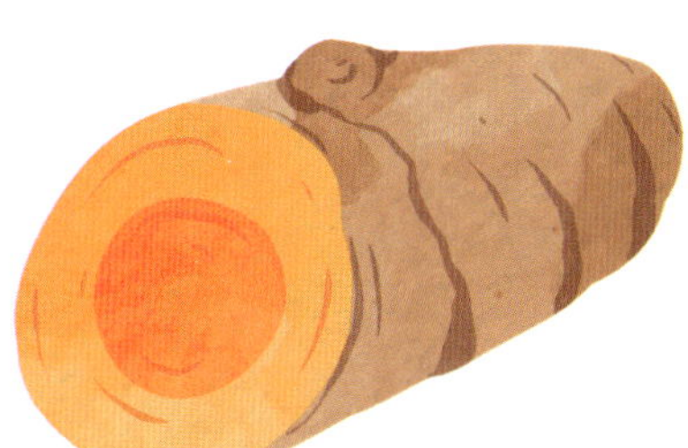

CHAPTER 11

# NAVIGATING THE MEDITERRANEAN PATH, SHOPPING SMARTS AND MEAL PLANNING

Now for the fun part. Are you ready to learn how to create personalised, budget-friendly, Mediterranean-style anti-inflammatory meals? Having explored the science behind anti-inflammatory nutrition, it's time to bridge the gap between research and your dinner plate. Every meal is a molecular messenger, influencing your immune response, gut health and brain function. Every bite is thus an opportunity to fight inflammation or fuel it.

In this chapter, you'll discover my road MAP to better health – the classic Mediterranean diet supercharged with inflammation-fighting foods. I'll guide you through the simple '4-3-2-1' plate method, provide sample meal ideas and shopping lists, plus strategies for overcoming common challenges. Whether you're new to anti-inflammatory eating or ready to elevate your current approach, you'll find steps to transform your kitchen into an inflammation-calming command centre.

For centuries, the culinary traditions of countries bordering the Mediterranean Sea have prioritised fresh, whole foods over processed ones. This approach is not only delicious but is also recognised as one of the world's most powerful anti-inflammatory diets.

Scientific interest in the diet grew in the 1950s, when researchers observed that people in Mediterranean regions had significantly lower rates of heart disease than those in the USA and northern Europe. This led to Dr Ancel Keys's landmark 'Seven Countries Study', which revealed that despite consuming dietary fats, people in Greece and Italy maintained better cardiovascular health. Their diet – rich in antioxidants, fibre and healthy fats (primarily from olive oil, nuts and fish) – was found to play a key role in reducing inflammation. The traditional Mediterranean lifestyle, which emphasises social and mindful eating, regular physical activity and stress reduction, also contributes to increased longevity and overall health.

The benefits of the Mediterranean diet have been confirmed by extensive modern research studies, linking it to reduced rates of heart disease, neurodegenerative conditions and chronic inflammation. For instance, a prominent study published in *The New England Journal of Medicine* found that individuals who followed a Mediterranean diet supplemented with extra nuts or olive oil had significantly lower markers of inflammation than those on a standard low-fat diet.

So why is the Mediterranean diet so effective? One major reason is the high levels of omega-3 fatty acids from fish. These essential fats help to lower levels of pro-inflammatory cytokines. Also, the diet's emphasis on fruits and vegetables means the body is flooded with antioxidants, which combat oxidative stress (the cellular equivalent of rusting). Extra virgin olive oil, a staple in Mediterranean cooking, contains polyphenols that actively fight inflammation. And let's not forget fibre (plentiful in whole grains, legumes and vegetables) that nourishes gut bacteria, leading to a healthier, more balanced immune system.

The secret to this way of eating? It's all in the togetherness. This plan isn't just about one magic ingredient; it's all the fibre, healthy fats, polyphenols, omega-3s and probiotics working in combination to reduce inflammation. See it as your roadmap to a healthier, more vibrant you as you navigate the world of anti-inflammatory nutrition and unlock a life full of energy.

## THE INFLAMMATION-FIGHTING STACK

Stack the odds in your favour. Combine omega-3s, curcumin and polyphenol-rich foods to create a powerful anti-inflammatory shield. This stack works synergistically to cool inflammation and protect your body from the inside out. Then increase your intake of colourful vegetables, fatty fish, olive oil, nuts, seeds and fermented foods.

If you're unsure of what you need to cut down, start by consuming less of these inflammatory foods:

- Processed meats (bacon, salami, sausages)
- Refined carbohydrates (white bread, pastries, cakes)
- Deep-fried foods and those cooked in vegetable seed oils
- Added sugars and sweetened beverages
- Ultra-processed snack foods with artificial additives
- Excessive amounts of red meat
- Foods containing trans fats
- Alcohol (especially in large quantities)

This straightforward approach will help you incorporate anti-inflammatory foods into your daily routine while gently crowding out the inflammatory ones to create sustainable changes.

## YOUR ROAD MAP TO ANTI-INFLAMMATORY SUCCESS

While traditional Mediterranean eating patterns have proven remarkably effective for reducing inflammation, with some additional strategies you can enhance these benefits even further. This is why I've developed MAP. This refined approach preserves everything valuable about traditional Mediterranean eating while incorporating cutting-edge nutritional science.

Worry not, I'm not introducing you to just another 'Grandma's olive oil' diet! MAP enhances the timeless benefits of the Mediterranean diet by upsizing the anti-inflammatory ratio of foods, emphasising gut health and incorporating a wider range of anti-inflammatory foods. This approach includes gut-friendly and potent foods such as fermented vegetables, kefir and microalgae. MAP prioritises colourful choices like berries, fatty fish, broccoli, avocados, green tea, and spices like turmeric and ginger, all celebrated for their inflammation-fighting prowess.

A key focus of MAP is reducing AGEs, harmful compounds that form when protein or fat combines with sugar in the bloodstream. To achieve this, this plan encourages gentle cooking methods that minimise AGE formation, while limiting overly processed and high-glycaemic foods. MAP also incorporates strategies to boost SPMs production: eating wild-caught fatty fish regularly, using high-quality extra virgin olive oil and a having a daily dose of walnuts.

To further amplify the anti-inflammatory benefits, MAP includes foods that activate the Nrf2 pathway, such as broccoli sprouts, rosemary and turmeric paired with black pepper. Including fresh pineapple and papaya provides natural enzymatic support.

### SCIENCE CONNECTION

For a deeper understanding of the advanced anti-inflammatory properties of compounds like SPMs, Nrf2 pathway activators and proteolytic enzymes, see Chapter 8, where we explore them in detail. By combining these advanced anti-inflammatory concepts with the proven benefits of the Mediterranean diet, my approach offers a comprehensive way for you to start supercharging your energy.

## YOUR PERFECT PLATE: Building the ultimate Mediterranean anti-inflammatory meal

Remember that old food pyramid nutritionists love to knock? I've flipped the script with my MAP approach. Instead of a pyramid, I use the 4-3-2-1 MAP plate method for a balanced meal. It's simple:

- 40% serve of vegetables
- 30% serve of lean protein
- 20% serve of whole grains
- 10% serve of healthy fats

This visual guide makes healthy eating a breeze! It's a balanced approach that ensures your diet is rich in antioxidants, fibre and essential nutrients for gut health.

# BUILD YOUR OWN MAP BOWL

Here's an example of how you could create your own MAP meal bowl, incorporating the principles of the plan.

## 40% vegetables and leafy greens

- Grilled zucchini (courgette), cucumber and rocket (arugula)
- Fermented vegetables like sauerkraut for gut health
- Broccoli sprouts for Nrf2 activation

## 30% lean proteins

- Grilled wild salmon with lemon and herbs (like rosemary for Nrf2 activation)
- Some cultured cheese or Greek yogurt for additional fermented protein sources

## 20% whole grains and starchy veggies

- Quinoa with chopped parsley and lemon zest
- Sweet potatoes or beetroot for added fibre and antioxidants

## 10% healthy fats

- Drizzle of extra virgin olive oil or linseed (flaxseed) oil
- Chopped walnuts for SPM production

## Additional touches

- Sprinkle some turmeric with black pepper on top for enhanced anti-inflammatory effects.

- Serve with a side of green tea or a small serving of berries for added antioxidants.

This meal combines the traditional Mediterranean diet with advanced anti-inflammatory strategies that promote good gut health, reduce AGEs and activate beneficial pathways like Nrf2. By using high-quality proteins and veggies, MAP enhances your gut, brain and immune health. It's a balanced eating plan that reduces inflammation without sacrificing flavour or flexibility.

## MAP MEAL MAGIC AND EASY TIPS FOR CREATING ANTI-INFLAMMATORY MEALS

Here are some tips to help you incorporate gut-healing foods into your MAP meals:

### Breakfast

- Make it nutrient-dense, protein-rich and anti-inflammatory.
- Include whole grains, fruits, nuts, eggs and fermented dairy.
- Examples: Greek yogurt or kefir with berries, walnuts; Turkish eggs with rocket & radish salad (page 143) or Salmon frittatas (page 147).

### Lunch

- Make it the largest meal, including vegetables and lean proteins.
- Use anti-inflammatory ingredients and Mediterranean staples.
- Examples: grain bowls with quinoa, roasted vegetables, wild-caught salmon and olive oil dressing; Polyphenol-rich power bowl with a side of sauerkraut (page 168)

## Dinner

- Make it early and lighter than lunch, focused on vegetables and modest protein.
- Include foods that activate the Nrf2 pathway and support gut health.
- Examples: grilled vegetables with small portions of herb-marinated fish or poultry; large Mediterranean-style salad with broccoli sprouts, and olive oil dressing.

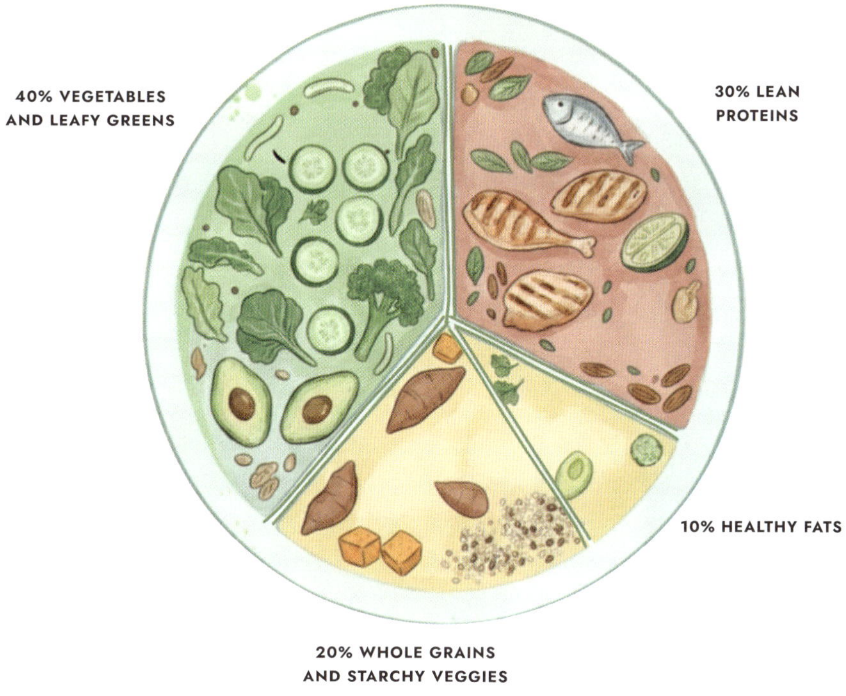

## Snacks

- Fresh fruits, especially berries
- Small handful of mixed nuts (walnuts work!)
- Vegetable crudités with hummus
- Goat's cheese and olives (occasionally)

## Portion perfection and how to fill your plate the MAP way

To ensure you're getting the right balance of nutrients, my MAP plate provides a simple guide for portion control. By dividing your plate into specific sections, you can easily manage your intake of vegetables, proteins, whole grains and healthy fats. Here's how to portion your meals effectively using easy-to-remember sizes – no need to turn your kitchen into a science laboratory. I've been there, done that all for you!

## Dividing your plate

- **Vegetables and leafy greens** = 40% of your plate. Imagine your plate is a clock face. Vegetables should cover a generous portion from 8 o'clock to 12 o'clock (about 40% of the plate).
- **Lean proteins** = 30% of your plate (palm-sized portion). Imagine a serve of protein as the size of your palm, fitting neatly in the centre.
- **Whole grains and starchy veggies** = 20% of your plate (fist-sized portion). Visualise this as the size of your clenched fist, providing a satisfying base for your meal.
- **Healthy fats** = 10% of your plate (1–2 tbsp extra virgin olive oil). Imagine this as a small dollop of olive oil or a small handful of nuts.

### Gut-healing foods to include

- At least one fermented food (Greek yogurt, cultured cheese, sauerkraut)
- At least 30 grams fibre from a variety of sources (vegetables, fruits, legumes, whole grains)
- Prebiotic-rich foods (garlic, onions, leeks, slightly green bananas, asparagus)
- Bone broth or collagen to support gut barrier integrity
- Foods that promote short-chain fatty acid production: resistant starch (cooked then cooled potatoes, green bananas), fibre-rich vegetables (broccoli, brussels sprouts) and whole grains (oats, quinoa)

Remember, this approach is about balance, not strict measurements. The social aspect of eating – sharing meals, eating slowly and enjoying mindfully – helps reduce stress and enhance the anti-inflammatory benefits of your diet.

## MADE JUST FOR YOU, CREATING A CUSTOM ANTI-INFLAMMATORY DIET

Research suggests that up to 60% of chronic diseases could be prevented by following a healthy, anti-inflammatory diet. But what works for one person may not work for another. Your genetic make-up, gut microbiome composition, stress levels and even your sleep patterns can influence how your body responds to certain foods.

Your individual responses to food can significantly influence inflammation. You can identify personal triggers through elimination diets or food sensitivity testing, which helps tailor dietary adjustments to your unique needs. You can also have a clinical nutritional consult with me: lee@superchareg‌dfood.com

## ONE-DAY MEDITERRANEAN ANTI-INFLAMMATORY MEAL PLAN

Let's look at what a day of eating might look like when following my MAP approach:

### UPON WAKING

- 1 glass warm water with fresh lemon juice and a thin slice of ginger
- Breakfast (7–8 am)
- Golden chia pudding
- 1 small handful blueberries
- Sprinkle of walnuts or linseeds (flaxseeds)
- 1 cup green tea or herbal tea
- Small serving of kefir or Greek yogurt

### MID-MORNING SNACK (10–11 AM)

- 1 small apple
- 1 tbsp almond butter
- Sprinkle of chia seeds
- Sparkling water with cucumber slices

### LUNCH (1–2 PM)

- Polyphenol-rich power bowl (page 168)
- Base: ½ cup quinoa
- Protein: 3–4 oz grilled wild salmon (quinoa for vegetarians)
- Vegetables: 1 cup rocket (arugula), ½ avocado, ¼ cup grated beetroot, ¼ cup shredded purple cabbage
- Toppings: 1 tbsp pumpkin seeds (pepitas), 2 tsp extra virgin olive oil, fresh lemon juice, pinch of sea salt
- Small side of fermented vegetables
- 1 cup herbal tea

## AFTERNOON SNACK (4–5 PM)

- Golden energy balls (page 229)
- Handful of almonds or walnuts
- 1 cup herbal tea

## DINNER (6–7 PM)

- Caper-crusted salmon with whipped Greek yogurt (page 199), or make it vegetarian with Soba noodles with zucchini & mango (page 215)
- Small side salad with lemon-olive oil dressing
- Small side of olives, cultured cheese or Greek yogurt
- 1 glass water with fresh mint

## EVENING (IF HUNGRY, 8–9 PM)

- ½ cup coconut yogurt with cinnamon
- Small handful of walnuts
- 1 cup chamomile tea

## HYDRATION THROUGHOUT THE DAY

- 35 ml water for every kilogram of body weight

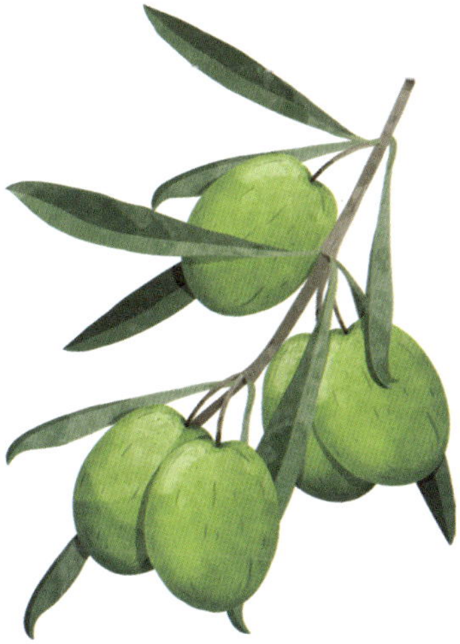

## FROM NOW TO WOW: Transitioning to your anti-inflammatory lifestyle

Shifting to a MAP approach doesn't happen overnight. Sustainable change comes from gradual, consistent adjustments that eventually become your new normal. Here's a structured approach to help you transition successfully.

Begin your journey by adding inflammation-fighting foods before removing anything from your diet. Incorporate fatty fish like salmon or mackerel weekly; add an extra serving of vibrant capsicums (peppers), leafy greens or purple carrots to dinner; and start each day with warm lemon water. Introduce fermented foods such as Greek yogurt, cultured cheese or fermented olives, and liberally use turmeric, ginger and oregano in your cooking. Like adding herbs to your garden, these small additions will flourish over time!

Next focus on swaps: extra virgin olive oil for refined seed oils, wholegrains for white carbs, and almonds or fresh berries for processed snacks. Replace a beef or pork meal with a chickpea, lentil or bean dish, and trade fizzy drinks (sodas) for herbal teas or cucumber-infused water. Once you've done this, mindfully reduce your inflammatory elements: halving your processed meat intake, baking or steaming foods instead of frying them, and becoming a nutrition label detective to spot hidden sugars and additives.

Finally, fine-tune your approach: experiment with Mediterranean recipes, roast vegetables to bring out their natural sweetness, and practise mindful eating at least once daily, putting down your phone and savouring each bite.

These small steps might seem modest on their own, but like the Mediterranean Sea itself, they create powerful waves of change!

### MEDITERRANEAN MAGIC:
### A delicious prescription

The Mediterranean diet's abundance of healthy fats, fibre and antioxidants reduces inflammation, supports brain health and energises your cells – delivering all three pillars in every meal.

## MAP ON A BUDGET: Eating healthy without breaking the bank

Eating to reduce inflammation doesn't have to break the bank. Here are practical strategies for keeping costs manageable.

### Prioritise investment foods

- Spend more on high-quality extra virgin olive oil, wild-caught fish and organic berries when possible.
- Save on other items so your total budget stays balanced.
- Remember, a small amount of high-quality MAP foods often provides more satisfaction and nutrition than larger amounts of lower-quality options.

### Smart shopping strategies

- Buy frozen fruits and vegetables, which are equally nutritious and often more affordable.
- Purchase seasonal produce when it's abundant and least expensive.
- Explore local farmers' markets, especially near closing time when vendors may discount their remaining items.

- Buy dry goods like legumes and grains in bulk.
- Grow anti-inflammatory herbs on your windowsill (basil, mint, rosemary, thyme).
- Shop the perimeter of the supermarket where whole foods are located.

### Budget-friendly MAP staples

- Tinned sardines and mackerel are often more affordable than fresh fish.
- Eggs are a versatile, high-quality protein.
- Cabbage is incredibly nutrient-dense and long-lasting.
- Frozen berries are more economical than fresh, especially out of season.
- Small amounts of dried herbs and spices pack a powerful anti-inflammatory punch.
- Legumes like lentils and chickpeas (garbanzo beans) cost pennies per serving.
- Oats are versatile, filling and rich in anti-inflammatory compounds.

## TRACKING YOUR MAP PROGRESS

Consider keeping a journal to note changes in your energy levels, sleep quality, digestion, mood and specific symptoms as you follow the MAP approach. This becomes your personal record of improvement, especially on days when your motivation might waver. Many people are surprised to discover connections between certain foods and symptoms they hadn't previously linked to their eating patterns.

## GRADUAL CHANGES: Progress, not perfection

It's easy to feel overwhelmed when making dietary changes but remember: the goal is progress, not perfection. No one eats perfectly all the time. Even the healthiest Mediterranean grandmothers probably sneak a pastry now and then. The key is to consistently make better choices, one meal at a time.

By integrating anti-inflammatory foods into your diet and reducing inflammatory triggers, you can transform your health at the cellular level. Along with managing inflammation, this approach enhances your energy, supports brain function and strengthens immunity. And who doesn't want to feel like the best, most vibrant version of themselves?

So start where you are. Swap out that fizzy drink (soda) for green tea. Add an extra serving of vegetables to your dinner. Choose olive oil over margarine. Every little step adds up to big, lasting health benefits.

Remember these core principles:

- Add before you subtract, gradually introducing anti-inflammatory foods.
- Focus on quality ingredients, particularly for olive oil, fatty fish and produce.
- Listen to your body's unique responses and personalise accordingly.
- Approach the journey with patience – progress matters more than perfection.
- Use the comprehensive shopping list as your guide to stocking an anti-inflammatory kitchen.

By following the MAP approach, you're not just reducing inflammatory triggers but actively supporting your body's natural healing processes, enhancing your energy and building long-term health resilience. Every anti-inflammatory meal choice is an investment in your current and future well-being.

# YOUR SHOPPING LIST OF ANTI-INFLAMMATORY STAPLES

Armed with knowledge about the MAP approach, you're now ready to stock your kitchen. This is a comprehensive shopping list organised by category. It's your guide when navigating grocery stores or farmers' markets.

## How to stock your kitchen the anti-inflammatory way

Start gradually. You don't need to buy everything at once. Begin with the basics and build your anti-inflammatory pantry over time.

- **Prioritise quality.** It's better to have smaller amounts of high-quality ingredients than larger amounts of lower-quality options. Invest in good olive oil, fresh spices and quality proteins.
- **Shop seasonally.** Many items on this list will be more nutritious, flavourful and affordable when purchased in season.
- **Store ingredients properly.** Many anti-inflammatory ingredients like nuts, seeds and oils are rich in beneficial but delicate fats that can oxidise. Store them properly in airtight containers, away from heat and light.
- **Personalise your diet.** Remember that the most important aspect of an anti-inflammatory diet is how it works for your unique body. Pay attention to how you feel after eating certain foods and adjust your shopping list accordingly.

## Comprehensive MAP food list

Nature has provided us with an extraordinary pharmacy of anti-inflammatory foods that you don't need a prescription to access. From vibrant berries bursting with antioxidants to omega-3-rich fish that calm cellular chaos, your local supermarket is a treasure trove of healing ingredients. Flip to Appendix 1 at the back of this book for your comprehensive guide to stocking an inflammation-fighting kitchen.

Here's to your MAP journey – may it be filled with delicious meals, improved energy and vibrant health for years to come!

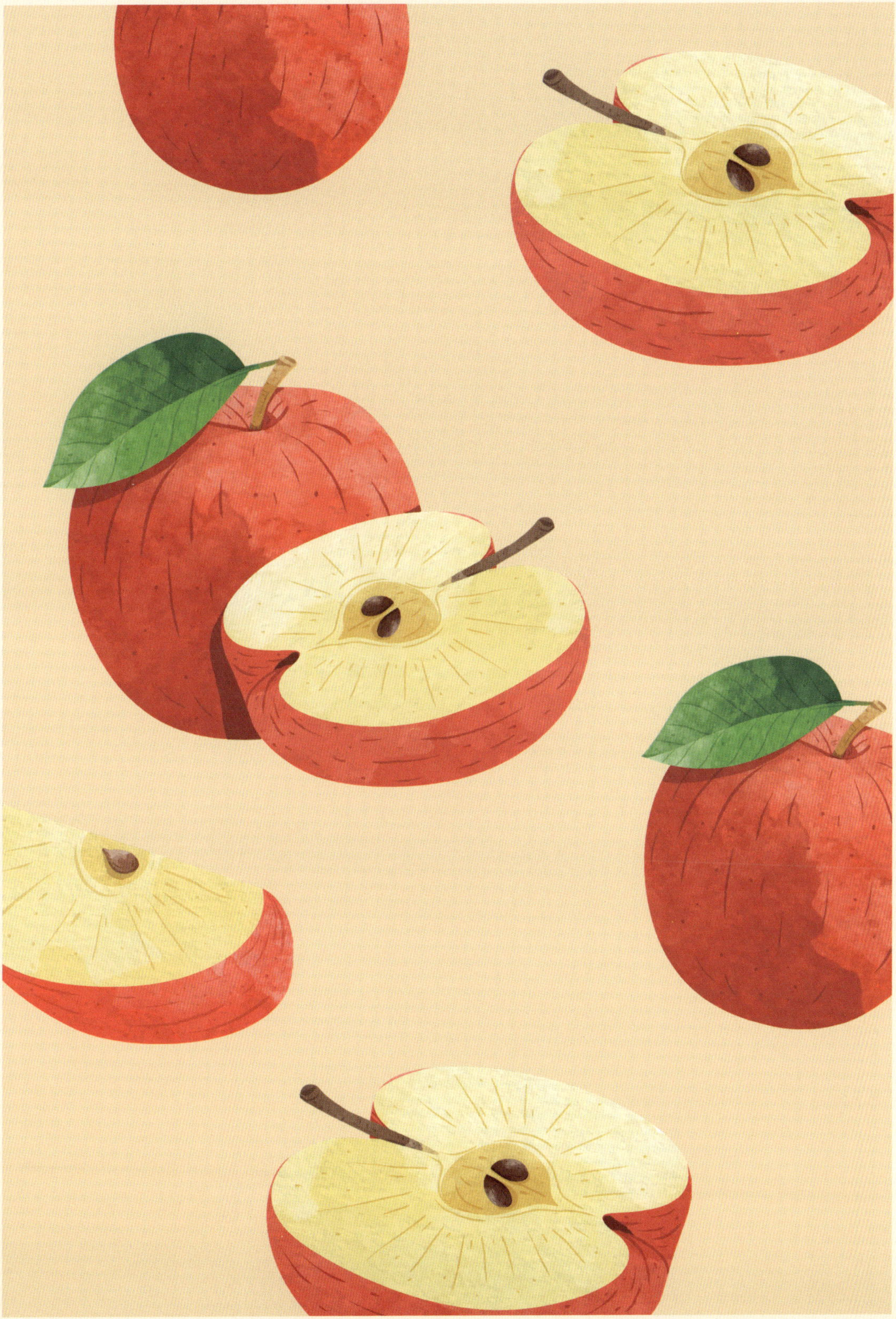

CHAPTER 12

# EAT TO HEAL WITH 60 DELICIOUS ANTI-INFLAMMATORY RECIPES

# RECIPE KEY: The three pillars of healing food

In *Eat to Heal*, each recipe has been lovingly crafted to serve one of your body's vital healing systems. The following icons next to each dish represent the three foundational pillars of this anti-inflammatory approach to eating.

## Anti-inflammatory champions

These are your heavy-hitters against inflammation – think turmeric, ginger, polyphenols, cruciferous vegetables and gut-healing ingredients. These recipes help to calm chronic inflammation, restore balance and protect against disease.

*These are your inner fire extinguishers.*

## Nervous system nurturers

Designed to nourish your brain and calm your nervous system, these meals are rich in omega-3s, B vitamins, magnesium and amino acids. They support neurotransmitter production, vagal tone, and help reduce stress and anxiety.

*These bring more calm, clarity and connection to your day.*

## Cellular energy boosters

These recipes are like rocket fuel for your mitochondria. Packed with complex carbs, quality protein, antioxidants and key nutrients like CoQ10 and iron, they're designed to energise your cells, boost your metabolism, and keep you vibrant and vital.

*Think power, stamina and sustained energy.*

The beauty of these pillars is how they overlap. Many recipes support multiple systems – that's the magic of whole food nutrition. Each meal contains nutrients working in harmony to support your body's innate healing. The icon guides indicate the recipe's main healing pillar – enjoy mixing and matching their anti-inflammatory, nervous system-nourishing and energy-boosting benefits in your own meal plans.

# 7 DAYS OF DELICIOUS ANTI-INFLAMMATORY MEALS

| DAY | BREAKFAST | LUNCH | DINNER | DESSERTS, SNACKS AND SAVOURIES |
|---|---|---|---|---|
| MON | Turkish eggs with rocket & radish salad (p. 143) | Black bean taco bowl with tahini dressing (p. 174) | Caper-crusted salmon with whipped Greek yogurt (p. 199) | Golden energy balls (p. 229) |
| TUE | Anti-inflammatory smoothie bowl (p. 146) | Air fryer salmon with dressed-up greens (p. 165) | Turmeric-spiced chicken with herb sauce (p. 197) | Feta & melon mosaic with maple pistachios (p. 237) |
| WED | Salmon frittatas (p. 147) | Roasted vegetable salad (p. 167) | Barley & roasted carrot risotto (p. 221) | Sardine crackers (p. 230) |
| THUR | Ginger quinoa breakfast porridge (p. 148) | Polyphenol-rich power bowl (p. 168) | Cauliflower steaks with za'atar (p. 203) | Almond-cacao crunch bark with hemp seeds (p. 239) |
| FRI | Blueberry antioxident overnight oats (p. 149) | Omega-rich mackerel niçoise salad (p. 169) | Sardine, zucchini & pea fritters with mint yogurt (p. 223) | Lemon & olive oil ice cream (p. 243) |
| SAT | Greek sheet-pan eggs with herbs & feta (p. 153) | Cucumber rolls with smoked trout (p. 177) | Low & slow bone broth stew (p. 207) | Raspberry-pistachio rocky-road bars (p. 235) |
| SUN | Buckwheat banana crêpes with figs & fresh berries (p. 159) | Tempeh, olive & feta skewers (p. 183) | Smoked trout frittata with pesto & salad (p. 205) | Inflammation-fighting trail mix (p. 228) |

# 60 MAP RECIPES TO BOOST YOUR ANTI-INFLAMMATORY LIFESTYLE

## ABOUT THE RECIPES

These recipes are designed to be easy, nutrient-dense and anti-inflammatory to support a balanced diet. Enjoy experimenting with the textures and flavours of these wholesome meals!

## MEAL PREP TIPS:

- Batch-cook proteins like salmon and chicken for easy lunches.
- Make extra frittatas, trail mix and smoothies for grab-and-go snacks.
- Use leftovers creatively (such as salmon for salads, roasted vegetables for bowls).
- Chop and store vegetables in advance to save time during the week.
- Make a big batch of bone broth to use as a base for soups and stews.
- Pre-portion smoothie ingredients in freezer bags for quick blending.
- Prepare spice blends and dressings in jars for easy seasoning.

## A NOTE ABOUT THE MEASUREMENTS

Please note that the cup and spoon measures in these recipes are based on Australian sizes. (The USA and UK use 15 ml tablespoon measures.)

- 1 cup = 250 ml or 8½ fl oz
- 1 tablespoon = 20 ml or ⅔ fl oz

Oven temperatures given are for conventional ovens.

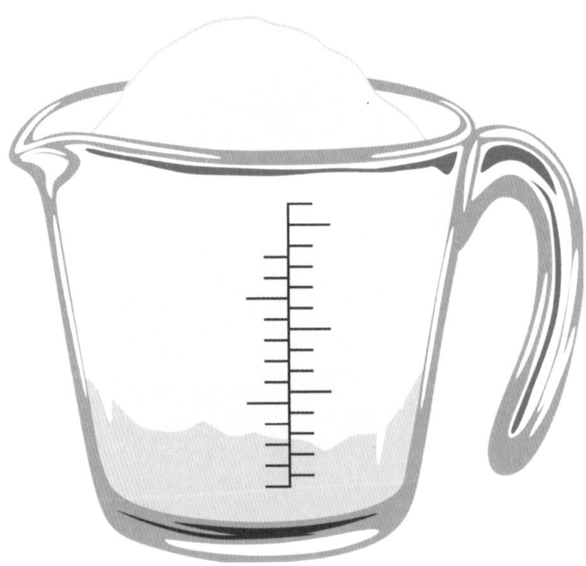

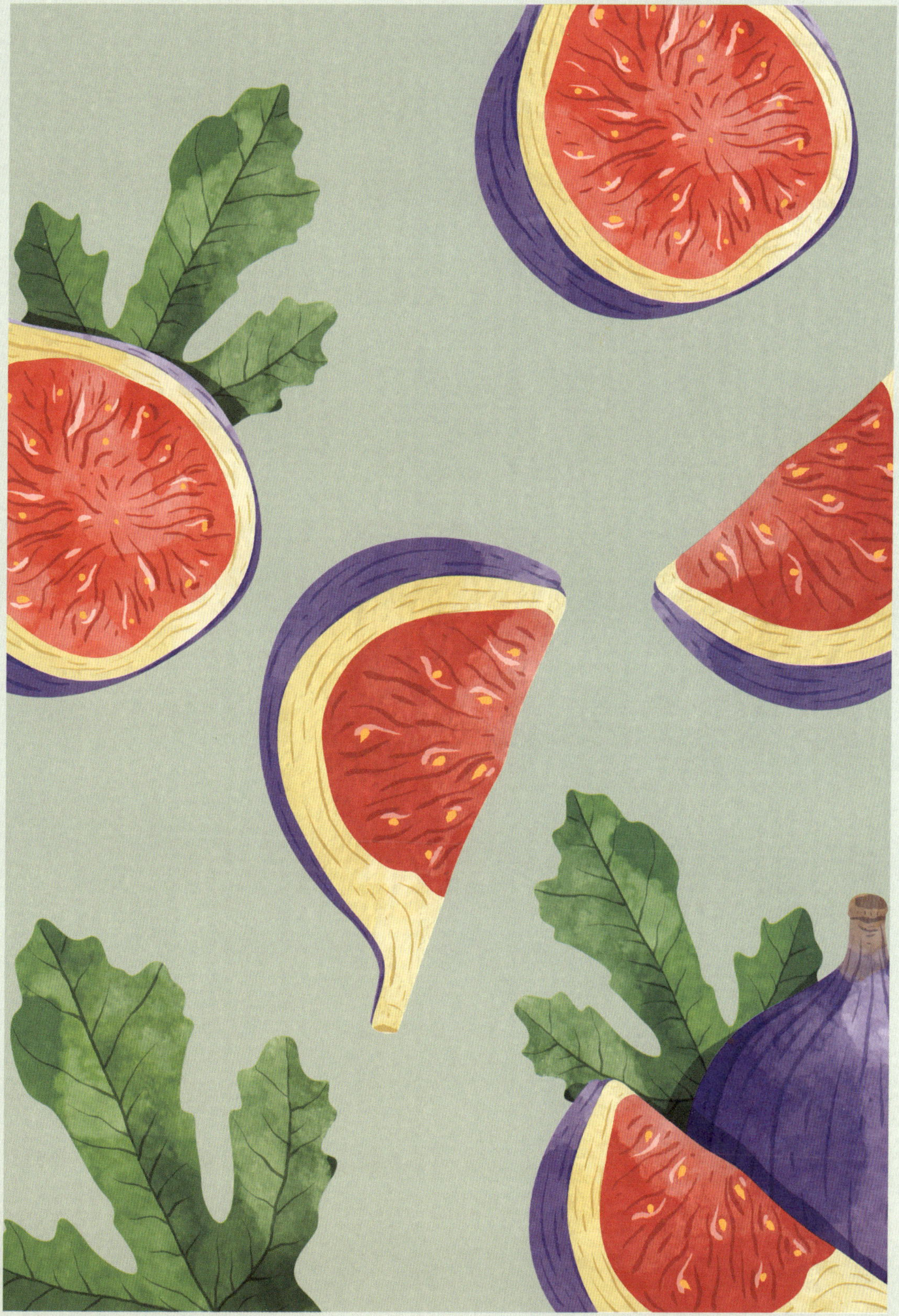

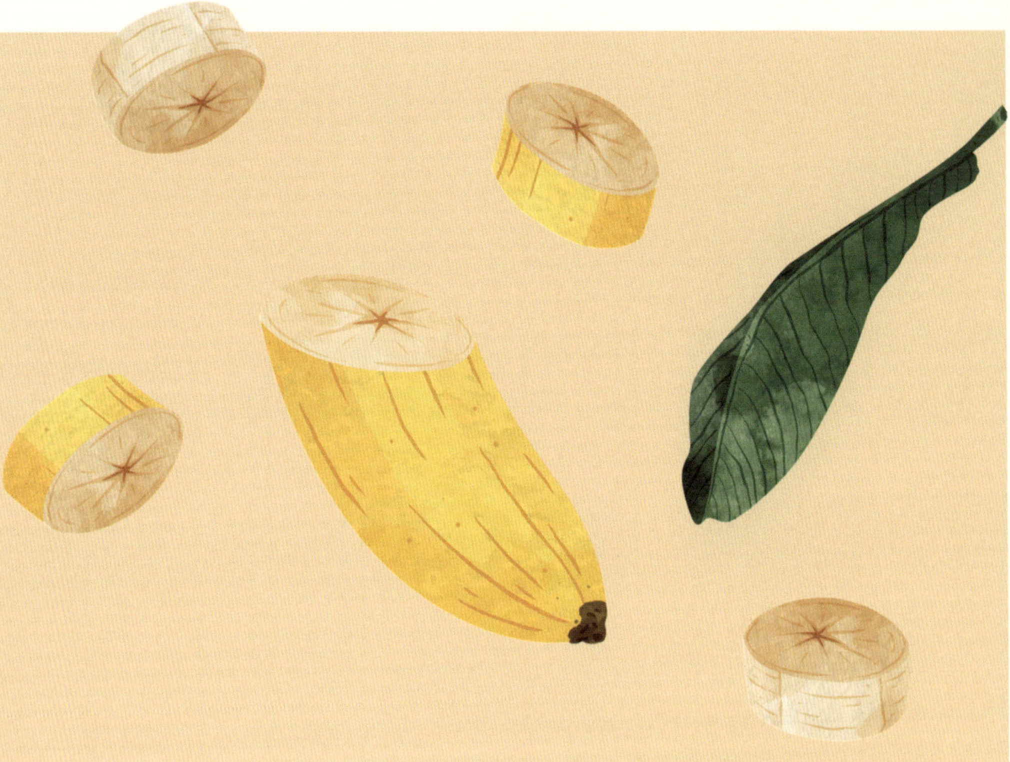

# BREAKFASTS

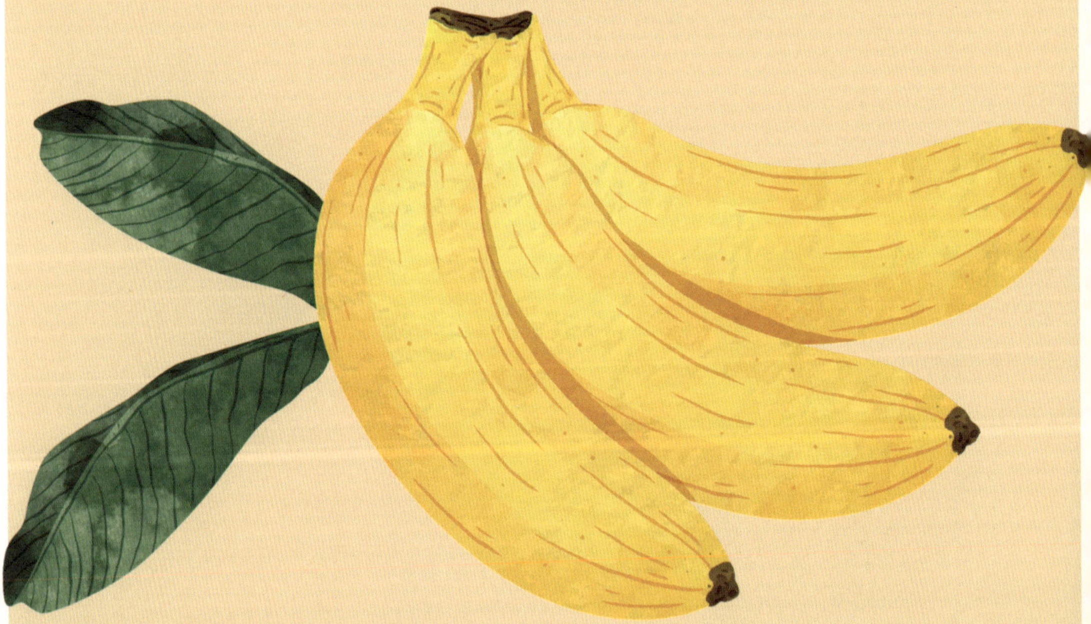

# TURKISH EGGS WITH ROCKET & RADISH SALAD

Your mitochondria will get a serious energy upgrade with this Mediterranean beauty that transforms simple eggs into cellular fuel. The silky poached eggs deliver complete protein for muscle recovery, while the tangy Greek yogurt provides probiotics and extra protein for sustained stamina. Peppery rocket (arugula) is loaded with nitrates that help optimise cellular oxygen delivery, giving your cells their own oxygen express lane.

**Serves 2**

## INGREDIENTS

4 tbsp Greek yogurt

1 clove garlic, minced

2 tbsp lemon juice

Sea salt and freshly ground black pepper

2 eggs

Handful of rocket (arugula)

½ avocado, roughly chopped

4 radishes, sliced thinly

1 tbsp extra virgin olive oil

2 tbsp Spiced nut & seed dukkah sprinkle (page 248)

## METHOD

Mix the yogurt with the garlic, lemon juice, and salt and pepper to taste. Set aside.

Bring a large pot of water to a gentle simmer. Add a generous amount of salt.

Crack each egg into a fine mesh strainer to remove excess loose whites then place into separate cups. Once the water is simmering, stir in a circular motion to create a whirlpool then carefully drop each egg into the water. Turn off the heat and let sit for 4–5 minutes.

Remove eggs with a slotted spoon.

Smear the yogurt on a plate or shallow bowl and top with the rocket, avocado pieces and radish slices. Add an egg on top then drizzle with olive oil, a pinch of salt and pepper, and dukkah.

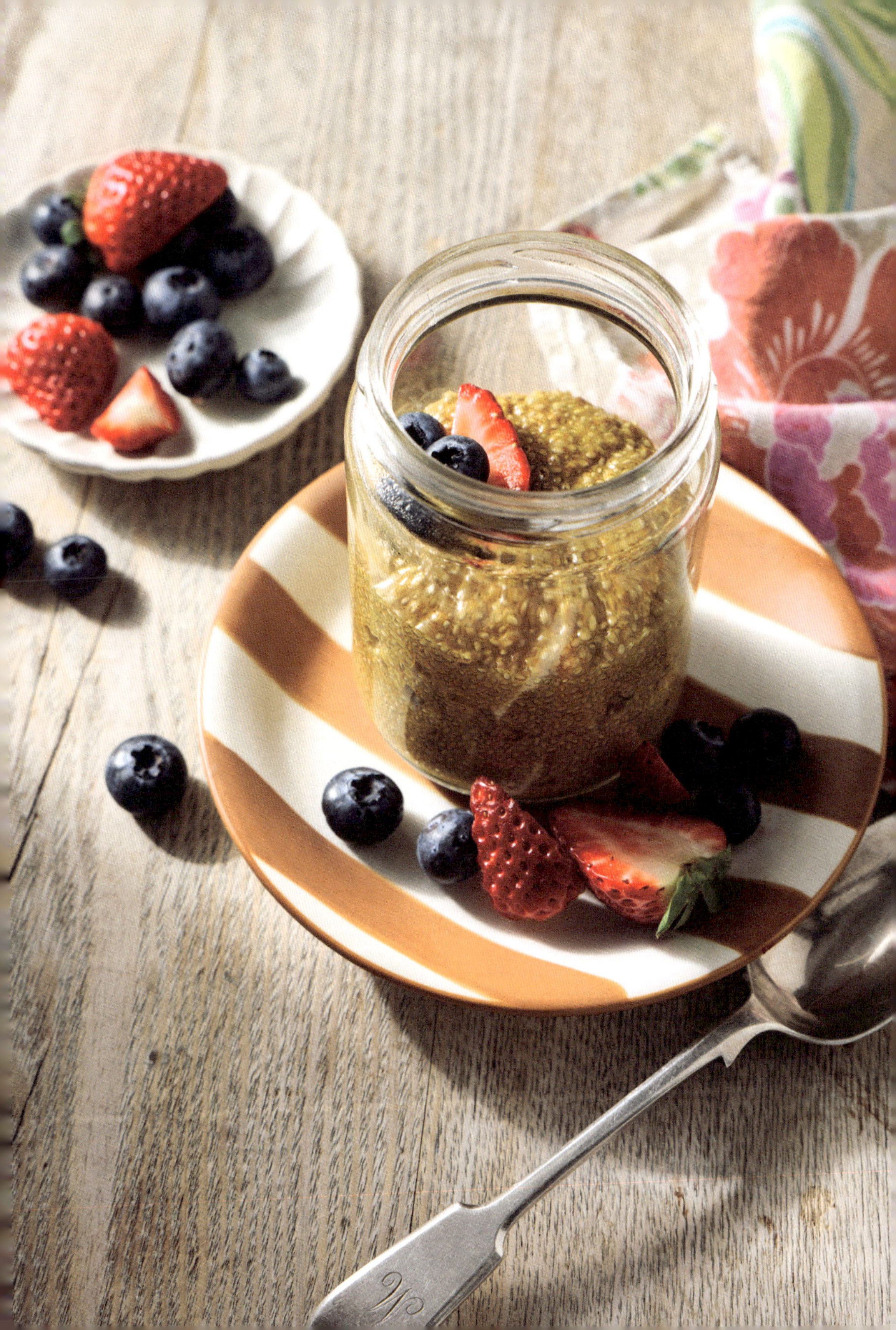

# GOLDEN CHIA PUDDING

This creamy and nutrient-dense pudding is packed with anti-inflammatory turmeric and omega-3-rich chia seeds. The combination of healthy fats, fibre and antioxidants supports digestion while keeping blood glucose stable.

**Serves 2**

### INGREDIENTS

4 tbsp chia seeds
⅔ cup coconut milk
1 tbsp raw yacon or maple syrup
½ tsp ground cinnamon
½ tsp ground turmeric
½ tsp vanilla extract
¼ cup fresh berries
2 tbsp crushed walnuts (optional)

### METHOD

In a large jar (or two small individual jars if you don't want to share) mix the chia seeds with the coconut milk, yacon syrup, cinnamon, turmeric and vanilla. Stir well or shake to combine. Refrigerate overnight, stirring once after 30 minutes to prevent clumping.

Serve chilled, topped with berries and walnuts.

# ANTI-INFLAMMATORY SMOOTHIE BOWL

My vibrant smoothie bowl is loaded with antioxidants from blueberries and polyphenols from spinach, helping to reduce inflammation and support brain health. The fibre content aids digestion, while avocado and linseeds (flaxseeds) provide healthy fats for long-lasting energy.

***Cooking tip:*** *Using frozen banana gives a creamier texture.*

**Serves 1**

## INGREDIENTS

½ cup frozen wild blueberries

½ frozen banana

½ cup spinach

½ avocado

1 tbsp linseeds (flaxseeds)

½ cup coconut yogurt

½ cup almond milk

1 tbsp hemp seeds, for topping

1 tbsp shredded coconut, for topping

## METHOD

Blend all the ingredients except hemp seeds and coconut until smooth. Pour into a bowl and top with the hemp seeds and shredded coconut.

# SALMON FRITTATAS

These protein-packed frittatas contain wild salmon, a rich source of omega-3 fatty acids that help support brain function. The combination of eggs, spinach and turmeric promotes gut health and cellular repair. They taste really lovely with goat's cheese.

***Cooking tip:*** *Let the frittatas cool slightly before removing them from the tins for easy release.*

**Serves 3 (2 frittatas each)**

## INGREDIENTS

- 5 eggs
- ½ cup cooked wild salmon, flaked (or canned salmon)
- ¼ cup chopped baby spinach
- 2 spring onions (scallions), chopped
- ½ tsp ground turmeric
- ¼ tsp freshly ground black pepper
- 1 tbsp extra virgin olive oil
- ½ cup crumbled goat's cheese (optional)

## METHOD

Preheat the oven to 180°C (350°F). Line a 6-cup muffin tin with paper liners.

Whisk the eggs and mix in the salmon, spinach, spring onions, turmeric, pepper and olive oil. Pour into the lined muffin tins and add goat's cheese (if using). Bake for 15–20 minutes or until set.

Let cool slightly before removing from tins.

# GINGER QUINOA BREAKFAST PORRIDGE

A warming and gut-friendly porridge that's rich in anti-inflammatory ginger and fibre-packed quinoa. This dish helps regulate your digestion while providing a steady release of energy throughout the morning.

***Cooking tip:*** *Toast the quinoa lightly before adding the liquid to enhance its nutty flavour.*

**Serves 2**

## INGREDIENTS

½ cup uncooked quinoa, rinsed
1 cup coconut or almond milk
1 tsp grated fresh ginger
½ tsp ground cinnamon
½ tsp vanilla extract
¼ tsp lemon zest
Pinch of salt
1 tbsp linseeds (flaxseeds)
1 tsp monk fruit sweetener, or maple or date syrup

*TOPPINGS*

Blueberries
Pumpkin seeds (pepitas)
Pomegranate seeds
Apple slices
Banana slices
Walnuts

## METHOD

Lightly toast the quinoa in a dry pot over medium heat for 2 minutes until fragrant. Add the coconut milk, ginger, cinnamon, vanilla, lemon zest and salt. Bring to a gentle simmer.

Reduce heat and cook for 10–12 minutes, stirring occasionally, until the quinoa is tender and the mixture thickens.

Stir in linseeds and sweetener. Serve warm with your choice of toppings.

# BLUEBERRY ANTIOXIDANT OVERNIGHT OATS

My creamy and indulgent overnight oats are rich in antioxidants, fibre and healthy fats. Blueberries provide a natural sweetness and a polyphenol boost, while shaved dark chocolate adds a decadent touch with anti-inflammatory flavonoids. Chia seeds and walnuts contribute essential omega-3 fatty acids, supporting brain health and reducing oxidative stress.

***Cooking tip:*** *Use a high-quality dark chocolate (85% cacao or higher) for maximum benefits.*

**Serves 1**

## INGREDIENTS

- ½ cup gluten-free oats
- 1 tbsp chia seeds
- ¼ cup coconut yogurt
- ½ cup almond milk
- 1 tsp monk fruit sweetener or maple syrup
- ½ tsp vanilla extract
- ½ tsp ground cinnamon
- ¼ cup blueberries
- 1 tbsp crushed walnuts
- 1 tbsp shaved dark chocolate (85% cacao or higher)
- 1 tbsp shredded coconut (optional)

## METHOD

Combine the oats, chia seeds, coconut yogurt, almond milk, sweetener, vanilla and cinnamon in a jar. Mix well and refrigerate overnight.

Serve chilled, topped with blueberries, walnuts, chocolate and coconut (if using).

# HEALING MUSHROOM & SPINACH EGG SCRAMBLE

A high-protein breakfast filled with antioxidants from mushrooms and iron-rich spinach. This dish supports brain function and immune health, and reduces inflammation. The addition of garlic, onion and fresh herbs enhances its depth of flavour, while an optional sprinkle of goat's cheese provides a creamy, tangy finish.

***Cooking tip:*** *Sauté mushrooms separately before adding eggs to enhance their flavour.*

**Serves 2**

## INGREDIENTS

1 tsp extra virgin olive oil

½ cup sliced shiitake mushrooms

1 clove garlic, minced

2 tbsp finely chopped onion

4 large eggs, whisked

½ cup spinach

1 tbsp chopped fresh herbs (chives, thyme or basil)

Sea salt and freshly ground black pepper

1 tbsp crumbled goat's cheese (optional)

## METHOD

Sauté the mushrooms, garlic and onion in olive oil for 3 minutes until softened.

Add the eggs, spinach and fresh herbs, stirring until eggs are cooked through. Season with salt and pepper.

Top with crumbled goat's cheese (if using) and serve warm.

# INFLAMMATION-REDUCING RAINBOW JUICE

This vibrant juice is loaded with anti-inflammatory and detoxifying ingredients such as turmeric, beetroot and ginger. It supports your digestion, liver function and overall vitality.

***Cooking tip:*** *Drink fresh for maximum nutrient absorption.*

**Serves 2**

## INGREDIENTS

2 carrots
2 celery stalks
1 beetroot
½ cucumber
Juice of ½ lemon
1 tsp fresh turmeric, grated
1 tsp fresh ginger, grated

## METHOD

Juice all the ingredients and serve immediately.

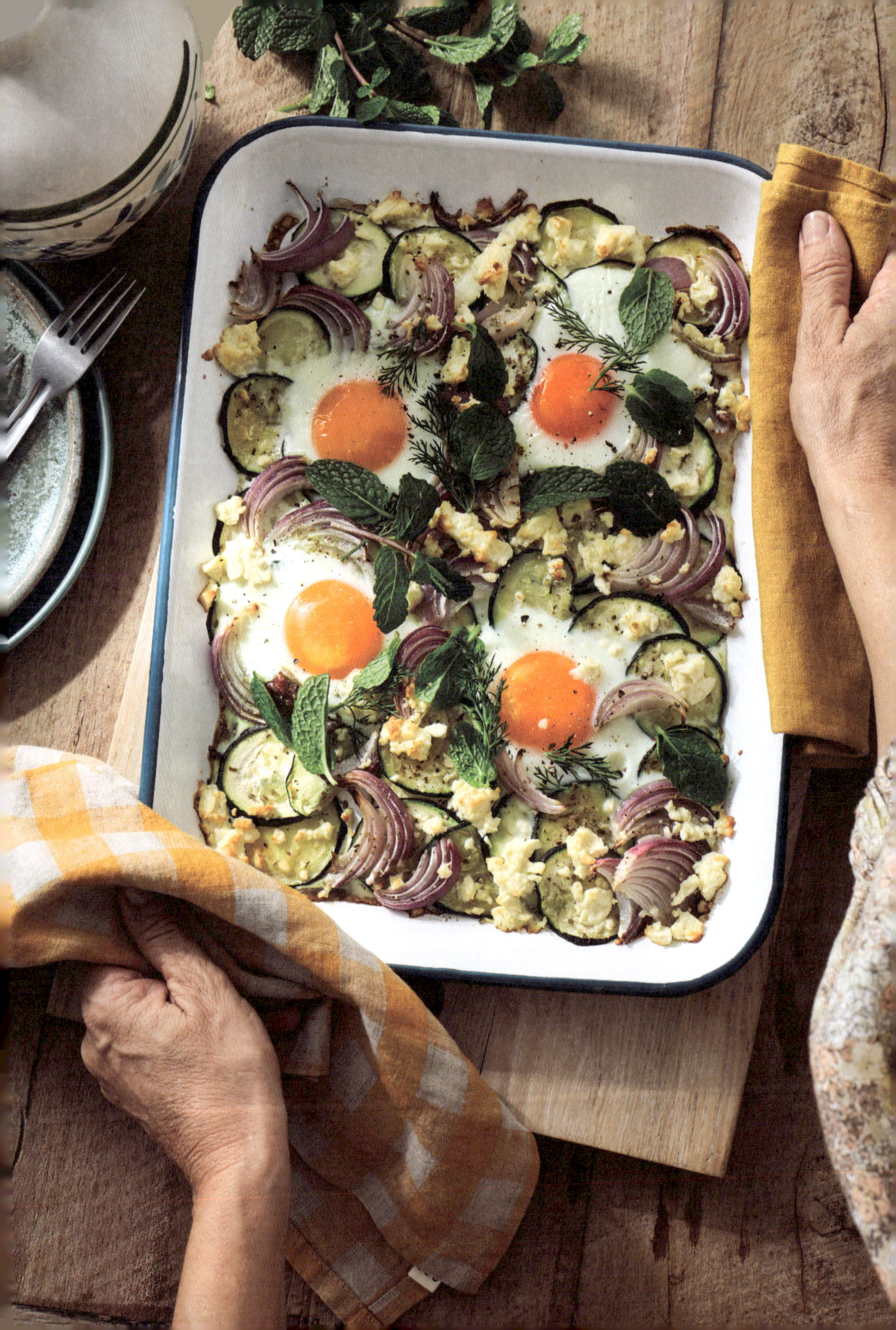

# GREEK SHEET-PAN EGGS WITH HERBS & FETA

This dish brings together everything great about a Mediterranean breakfast – flavourful herbs, creamy feta and softly roasted veg – all in one tray. Gently baking the eggs with zucchini (courgette), mint and dill keeps everything light and fresh while preserving the nutrients. It's an easy, fuss-free way to enjoy a protein-rich breakfast that delivers complete amino acids, essential B vitamins including B12 and folate, plus a satisfying sprinkle of omega-3s and magnesium with the seeds. The result is cellular fuel that supports your gut health, keeps inflammation low and provides sustained energy.

**Serves 4**

### INGREDIENTS

1 medium zucchini (courgette), thinly sliced

1 small red onion, finely sliced

1 tbsp extra virgin olive oil

1 tsp dried oregano

Sea salt and freshly ground black pepper

4 large pasture-raised eggs

60 g (2 oz) feta, crumbled

1 tbsp chopped fresh dill

1 tbsp chopped fresh mint

Sprinkle of hemp seeds or pumpkin seeds (pepitas) for topping (optional)

### METHOD

Preheat oven to 180°C (350°F). Line a baking tray with baking (parchment) paper.

Arrange the zucchini and red onion on the tray. Drizzle with olive oil and season with oregano, salt and pepper. Roast for 15 minutes until softened.

Remove from the oven, and gently create 4 small wells in the vegetables. Crack an egg into each well. Sprinkle over the feta. Return the dish to the oven and bake for another 8–10 minutes or until the eggs are just set.

Serve warm, garnished with the chopped fresh herbs and a sprinkle of seeds (if using).

# PROBIOTIC POWER BOWL WITH GREENS & AVOCADO

This savoury breakfast bowl is all about balance. It combines sautéed greens, crunchy cabbage, creamy avocado and probiotic-rich yogurt to help nourish the gut and keep you energised all morning. Quinoa provides slow-release energy and prebiotic fibre to support a diverse microbiome. A soft-boiled egg tops it off with high-quality protein, making this an ideal anti-inflammatory start to the day that's both satisfying and supportive of long-term gut health.

**Serves 2**

## INGREDIENTS

- 2 eggs
- 1 tsp extra virgin olive oil
- 2 big handfuls of mixed greens (kale, spinach or silverbeet/Swiss chard)
- ½ cup finely shredded red cabbage
- 1 tsp apple cider vinegar
- Pinch of sea salt
- ½ cup cooked quinoa
- 1 small avocado, sliced
- 4 tbsp natural sheep's or goat's yogurt
- Spiced nut & seed dukkah sprinkle (page 248)

## METHOD

Bring a small saucepan of water to the boil. Lower in the eggs and simmer for 6½ minutes. Transfer to cold water to stop the cooking.

In a frying pan, heat the olive oil over medium–low heat. Sauté the greens for 2–3 minutes until just wilted.

In a large bowl, massage the cabbage with apple cider vinegar and salt. Let it sit for 5 minutes.

Gently reheat or fluff the cooked quinoa if prepared in advance. Peel and halve the eggs.

To assemble, layer the quinoa, sautéed greens, cabbage, avocado and yogurt in individual bowls. Top with the eggs and a sprinkle of dukkah. Serve warm or at room temperature.

# EGG WRAP WITH GREENS, MUSHROOMS & LABNEH

This soft and savoury egg wrap is packed with colour and texture – perfect for anyone looking to upgrade their morning eggs. It's filled with sautéed asparagus, earthy mushrooms, wilted silverbeet (Swiss chard) and a generous spoonful of creamy labneh, all rolled into a light, omelette-style wrap. With gut-loving greens and naturally anti-inflammatory ingredients, it's a comforting yet functional start to the day that's easy on the digestive system and will supercharge your day.

**Serves 1**

## INGREDIENTS

- 1 tsp extra virgin olive oil
- 3 asparagus spears, chopped
- 3 chestnut mushrooms, sliced
- Handful of silverbeet (Swiss chard), roughly chopped
- 2 large eggs
- Sea salt and freshly ground black pepper
- 2 tbsp labneh

## METHOD

In a small frying pan, heat the olive oil and gently sauté the asparagus and mushrooms for 3–4 minutes. Add the silverbeet and cook for a further minute until just wilted. Remove the vegetables and set aside.

In a bowl, whisk the eggs with a pinch of salt and pepper. Pour into the same pan and cook on a low heat for 2–3 minutes until just set.

Spoon the cooked vegetables down the middle and add a dollop of labneh. Carefully fold over like a wrap and serve immediately.

# BAKED SWEET POTATO HASH BROWNS

These vibrant hash browns are a nutrient-dense twist on a comfort food classic. Sweet potatoes are rich in beta-carotene, a powerful antioxidant that supports your skin, vision and immune health. Chickpea (garbanzo bean) flour provides protein and fibre, while turmeric and cumin add anti-inflammatory benefits. Creamy avocado provides heart-healthy monounsaturated fats and potassium, and microgreens are a concentrated source of phytonutrients that support cellular health.

**Serves 2 (makes 4–6 small hash browns)**

## INGREDIENTS

*HASH BROWNS*

2 small or 1 large sweet potato, peeled and grated

2 tbsp chickpea (garbanzo bean) flour

1 tbsp extra virgin olive oil (plus more for brushing)

½ tsp ground cumin

¼ tsp ground turmeric

Sea salt and freshly ground black pepper

*SMASHED AVOCADO*

1 ripe avocado

Juice of ½ lemon

Pinch of sea salt

Freshly ground black pepper

*SALAD*

1 cup mixed microgreens

1 tsp extra virgin olive oil

Squeeze of lemon juice

Sea salt

*TOPPINGS*

1 tbsp hemp seeds, toasted pumpkin seeds (pepitas) or crushed walnuts

## METHOD

Preheat the oven to 180°C (350°F) and line a baking tray with baking (parchment) paper. Brush lightly with olive oil.

In a mixing bowl, combine the sweet potato, chickpea flour, olive oil, cumin, turmeric, salt and pepper. Mix well and let the mixture sit for 5–10 minutes to bind.

Scoop out portions and shape into small flat patties about 1 cm (½ inch) thick. Arrange on the prepared tray and brush the tops with a little more olive oil.

Bake for 25–30 minutes, flipping halfway, until golden brown and crisp around the edges. For extra crispness, increase the oven temperature to 200°C (390°F) for the final 5 minutes, watching carefully to prevent burning.

Meanwhile, smash the avocado with lemon juice, salt and pepper until creamy. In a separate bowl, toss the microgreens with olive oil, lemon juice and a pinch of salt.

Serve the warm hash browns topped with smashed avocado and the dressed microgreens. Sprinkle generously with your choice of seeds or nuts.

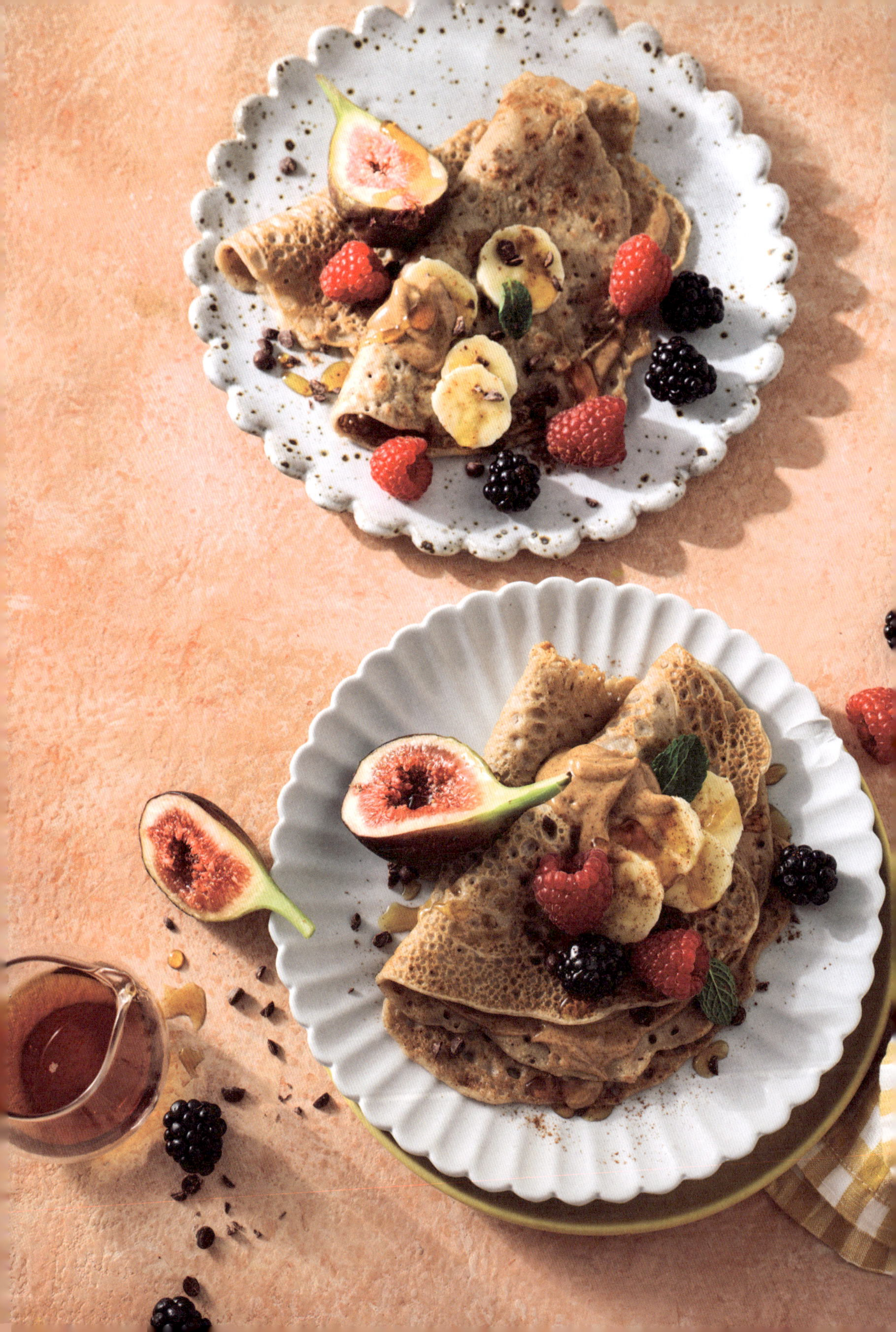

# BUCKWHEAT BANANA CRÊPES WITH FIGS & BERRIES

Light, nourishing and packed with gut-friendly resistant starch from just-ripe bananas, these naturally gluten-free buckwheat crêpes nourish your brain, calm your nervous system and support your digestive health and hormonal balance. Buckwheat is rich in rutin, which strengthens blood vessels. Figs and fresh berries add prebiotic fibre and polyphenols, while nut butter and cacao nibs provide healthy fats and antioxidants to support sustained energy and reduce inflammation.

**Serves 2 (makes 3–4 medium crêpes)**

## INGREDIENTS

*CRÊPES*

½ cup buckwheat flour

1 tsp ground linseeds (flaxseeds)

Sea salt

1 cup (250 ml/8½ fl oz) filtered water or unsweetened almond milk

Coconut oil, for cooking

*FILLING*

2 tbsp almond or walnut butter

1 slightly green banana, sliced

2 fresh figs, sliced (or 3 dried figs, softened in warm water)

½ cup fresh raspberries and blackberries

1 tsp cacao nibs

Drizzle of yacon syrup (optional)

Mint leaves (optional)

Pinch of cinnamon (optional)

## METHOD

In a bowl, whisk together the buckwheat flour, linseeds, salt and water (or almond milk) to make a thin batter. Let sit for 5–10 minutes to thicken slightly.

Heat a non-stick pan over medium heat with a little coconut oil. Pour in a ladleful of batter, swirling to coat the base. Cook for 2–3 minutes until the surface is dry and edges lift easily. Flip and cook for 1 minute more. Repeat with the remaining batter.

Spread each crêpe with nut butter, then layer with banana and fig slices and berries. Sprinkle with cacao nibs and a drizzle of yacon syrup, some mint leaves and a sprinkle of cinnamon (if using).

# HIGH-PROTEIN FRUIT SALAD

This vibrant fruit salad is a hydrating and energising way to start the day. Cottage cheese adds protein and beneficial probiotics to support muscle repair and gut health. Juicy watermelon, rockmelon (cantaloupe) and tangy passionfruit provide anti-inflammatory antioxidants and natural enzymes, while a sprinkle of pistachios offers healthy fats to keep blood glucose balanced. A nourishing option for warmer mornings, this recipe ticks every box of MAP – colourful, cooling and deeply supportive of cellular vitality.

**Serves 2**

## INGREDIENTS

1 cup full-fat cottage cheese
1 cup watermelon cubes
1 cup rockmelon (cantaloupe) cubes
1 passionfruit, halved
Zest and juice of ½ lime
1 tbsp chopped pistachios
1 tsp maple syrup (optional)

## METHOD

Divide the cottage cheese between two bowls. Top each bowl with cubes of watermelon and rockmelon. Spoon over the pulp from the passionfruit. Add a squeeze of lime juice and a little zest for brightness. Drizzle with maple syrup (if using). Sprinkle with pistachios for added crunch and anti-inflammatory fats.

Serve immediately while fresh and chilled.

# LUNCHES

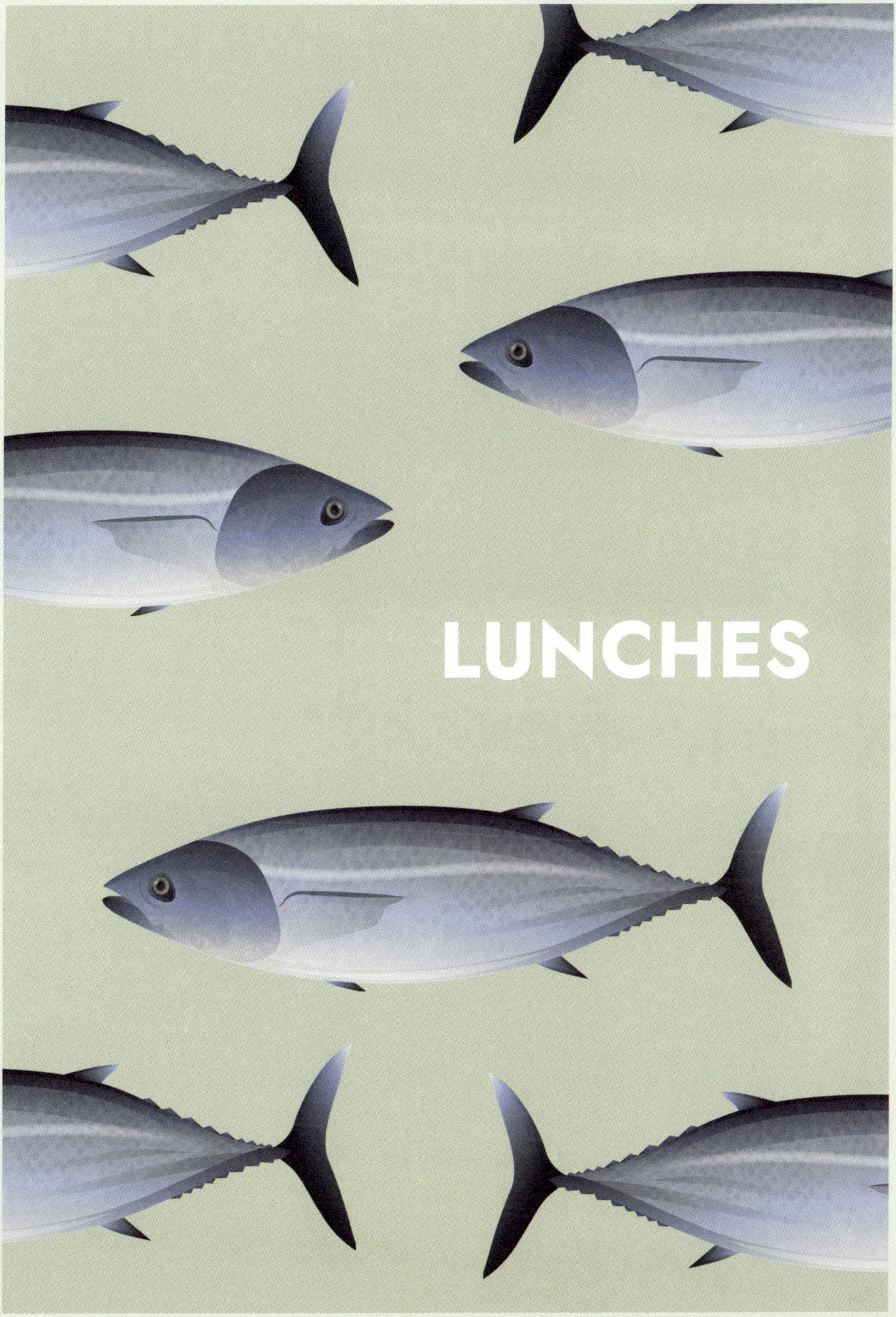

# CROWD-PLEASING FALAFEL SALAD WITH SHEEP'S YOGURT

***Cooking tip:*** *You can refrigerate any leftover falafels for a few days, or pop them in the freezer.*

**Serves 3 (makes 12 falafels)**

## INGREDIENTS

*HOMEMADE FALAFELS*

400 g (14 oz) black beans, cooked
400 g (14 oz) lentils, cooked
Bunch of fresh coriander (cilantro)
Juice of 1 lemon
2 tbsp sweet paprika
2 tbsp extra virgin olive oil
2 tbsp freshly ground black pepper
2 tbsp sea salt
1 heaped tbsp almond meal
1 heaped tsp ground turmeric

*SIDE SALAD*

6 cups mixed leaves
4 radishes, sliced
2 carrots, peeled and sliced
1 red onion, sliced
Handful of fresh mint
1 cup sheep's yogurt
4 tbsp almond butter (heated)
Extra virgin olive oil, for dressing
Freshly ground black pepper (optional)

## METHOD

To make the falafels, blend all the ingredients except almond meal in a food processor until combined. Stir in the almond meal slowly until it's just dry enough to handle. Scrape out the mixture and transfer to a bowl, cover and refrigerate for at least 1 hour or overnight.

Once chilled, use clean, wet hands to quickly divide and form the mixture into 12 falafels.

Preheat the oven to 175°C (345°F). Bake the felafels in the oven on a tray for 30 minutes or until golden. Remove from the oven and set aside.

To make the salad, arrange the salad ingredients in a large bowl and top with the sheep's yogurt and almond butter. Serve with falafels.

# CURCUMIN CAULIFLOWER RICE BOWL

A grain-free, anti-inflammatory bowl packed with fibre and potent anti-inflammatory turmeric. The cauliflower rice supports digestion and detoxification, while roasted crunchy chickpeas (garbanzo beans) add plant-based protein and a satisfying crunch. The garlic, onions and fresh herbs deepens the flavour profile, while toppings like toasted nuts, fresh lime and tahini drizzle provide extra layers of texture and taste.

### HOW TO MAKE CAULIFLOWER RICE:

**Food processor (fastest):** Cut cauliflower into florets. Pulse in food processor until it resembles rice (about 5–6 pulses). Don't overprocess or it becomes mushy.

**Box grater (no equipment):** Hold cauliflower by the stem. Grate using the medium-sized holes. Work over a large bowl to catch all the 'rice'.

***Cooking tip:*** *Lightly sauté the cauliflower rice to maintain its texture.*

**Serves 2**

### INGREDIENTS

*ROASTED CRUNCHY CHICKPEAS*

½ cup cooked chickpeas (garbanzo beans)
1 tsp extra virgin olive oil
¼ tsp ground coriander
¼ tsp ground cumin
Sea salt

*CAULIFLOWER RICE BOWL*

1 tbsp coconut oil
2 tbsp finely chopped onion
1 clove garlic, minced
1 cup riced cauliflower
½ tsp ground coriander
½ tsp ground cumin
½ tsp ground ginger
½ tsp ground turmeric
¼ tsp freshly ground black pepper
1 tbsp chopped fresh herbs (chives, thyme or basil)
1 tbsp chopped fresh coriander (cilantro)
1 tbsp toasted cashews or almonds
1 tbsp fresh lime juice
1 tbsp coconut flakes
1 tbsp tahini drizzle (optional)

### METHOD

To make the roasted chickpeas, preheat oven to 200°C (400°F). Toss the chickpeas with the olive oil, coriander, cumin and a pinch of salt. Roast for 20–25 minutes until crispy, shaking the pan halfway through. Set aside.

To make the cauliflower rice, heat the coconut oil in a frying pan and sauté the onions and garlic for 2 minutes.

Add the riced cauliflower, coriander, cumin, ginger, turmeric and pepper. Sauté for 3–4 minutes, stirring occasionally to make sure the rice does not get overcooked.

Stir in fresh herbs and roasted crunchy chickpeas. Serve warm, topped with fresh coriander, cashews or almonds, lime juice, coconut flakes and a drizzle of tahini (if using).

# AIR FRYER SALMON WITH DRESSED-UP GREENS

Designed to nourish your brain and calm your nervous system, this nutrient-dense meal is like a spa day for your neurons. The wild salmon delivers a hefty dose of omega-3s that support neurotransmitter production and reduce inflammation. The leafy kale provides folate and magnesium – essential minerals for maintaining healthy vagal tone and reducing stress. Those crunchy walnuts and linseed (flaxseed) oil are packed with alpha-linolenic acid (another omega-3) and vitamin E to protect your brain cells from oxidative stress. The creamy avocado brings healthy monounsaturated fats that help your body absorb all the brain-boosting nutrients. The dukkah seasoning adds a delicious Middle Eastern twist, plus extra magnesium and B vitamins from the nuts and seeds.

***Cooking tip:*** *Using an air fryer keeps the salmon crispy without needing excess oil.*

**Serves 2**

## INGREDIENTS

2 wild salmon fillets
1 tbsp extra virgin olive oil
1 tbsp dukkah
1 cup kale, washed and chopped
1 tbsp crushed walnuts
½ avocado, sliced
Sea salt and freshly ground black pepper

*DRESSING*

2 tbsp apple cider vinegar
2 tbsp lemon juice
2 tbsp linseed (flaxseed) oil
1 tsp Dijon mustard
1 tsp maple syrup

## METHOD

Pat dry the salmon fillets with a paper towel (kitchen paper). Rub with the olive oil and coat evenly with dukkah. Place the salmon in the air fryer and cook at 180°C (350°F) for 10–12 minutes.

Meanwhile, in a small bowl, whisk together all the dressing ingredients.

Toss the kale with the walnuts, avocado and dressing. Season with salt and pepper. Serve salmon on top of the dressed greens.

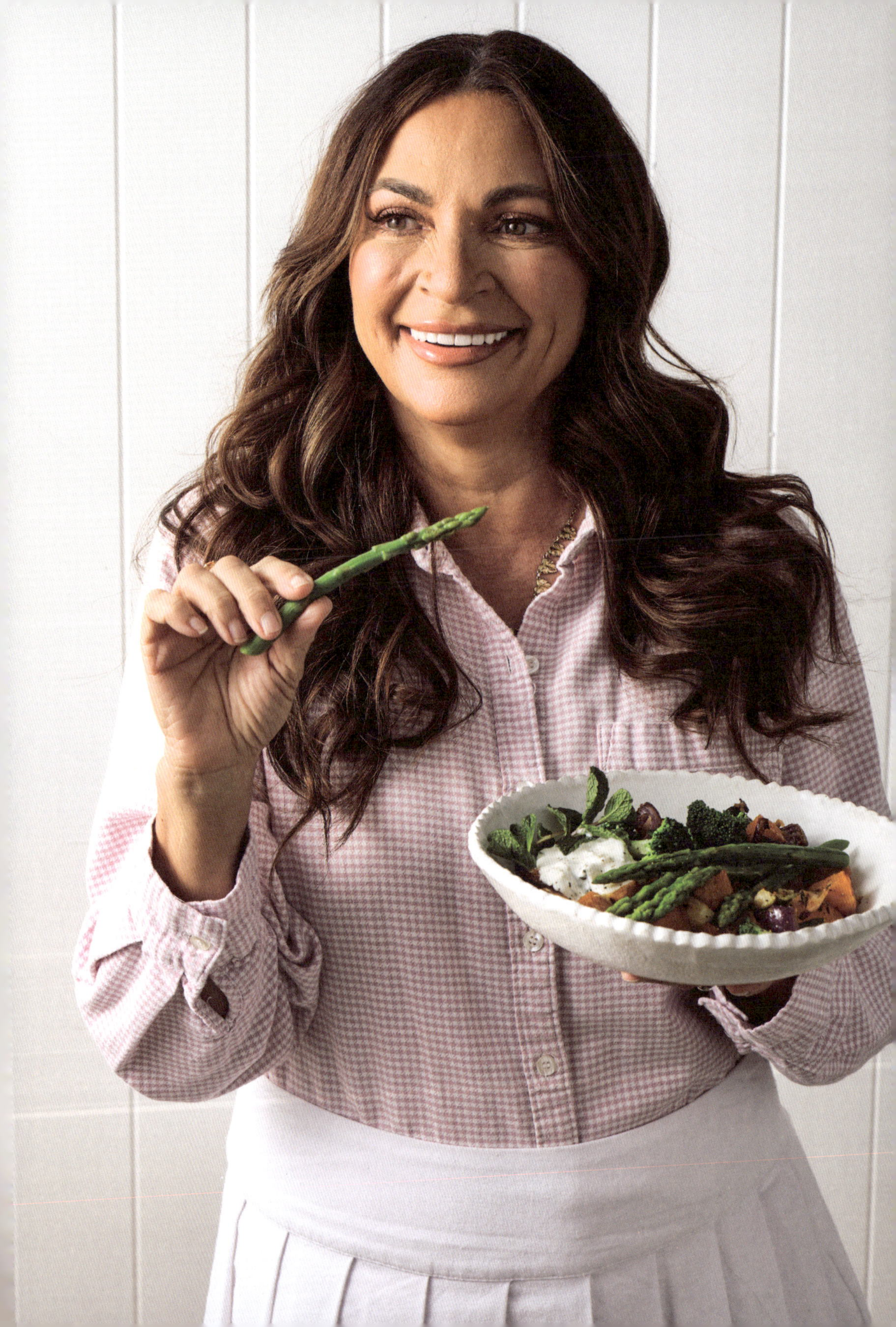

# ROASTED VEGETABLE SALAD

This dish helps fight oxidative stress while providing essential fibre and vitamins for gut health. The garlic, onions and fragrant herbs enhance the flavour and add anti-inflammatory benefits.

**Serves 3–4**

## INGREDIENTS

1 small sweet potato, diced

1 zucchini (courgette), chopped

1 cup broccoli florets

1 cup asparagus pieces, trimmed

1 small onion, sliced

3 cloves garlic, minced

2 tbsp extra virgin olive oil or avocado oil

1 tsp dried oregano

1 tsp smoked paprika

1 tsp fresh thyme leaves

2 tbsp apple cider vinegar

2 tbsp chopped fresh parsley or coriander (cilantro)

Sea salt and freshly ground black pepper

Dollop of tzatziki, to serve (optional)

Fresh mint leaves, to serve (optional)

## METHOD

Preheat the oven to 200°C (400°F) and line a baking tray with baking (parchment) paper. Place the baking tray in the oven while it preheats.

Pat dry the chopped vegetables with a paper towel (kitchen paper) to help them crisp up. In a bowl, toss the sweet potatoes, zucchini, onions and garlic with the olive oil, oregano, smoked paprika, thyme, salt and pepper. Spread vegetables onto the preheated baking tray, ensuring they are in a single layer and not overcrowded. Roast for 20 minutes, then toss the vegetables and sprinkle with apple cider vinegar. Roast for another 5–10 minutes.

While the vegetables are roasting, steam the broccoli and asparagus for about 3–4 minutes until tender but still vibrant.

Remove roasted vegetables from the oven and let them rest for a minute before transferring to a bowl.

Assemble the salad by combining the roasted and steamed vegetables. Sprinkle with fresh herbs and an extra pinch of salt and pepper. Add a dollop of tzatziki and mint leaves to serve (if using).

# POLYPHENOL-RICH POWER BOWL

Quinoa and chickpeas (garbanzo beans) deliver complex carbohydrates and complete proteins to keep your energy systems firing steadily, while those jewel-like pomegranate seeds and plump blueberries flood your cells with protective polyphenols. The creamy tahini dressing is loaded with magnesium, which your mitochondria need to produce ATP (your body's energy currency). The iron-rich kale and chickpeas help optimise oxygen delivery to your cells, while the slivered almonds add extra magnesium and healthy fats.

***Cooking tip:*** *Rinse quinoa before cooking to remove any bitterness.*

**Serves 2–3**

## INGREDIENTS

1 cup cooked quinoa
1 cup chopped kale
½ cup chickpeas (garbanzo beans)
½ cup blueberries
¼ cup slivered almonds
¼ cup crumbled feta
2 tbsp pomegranate seeds
2 tbsp extra virgin olive oil
Sea salt and freshly ground black pepper

*TAHINI DRESSING*

3 tbsp tahini
1 ½ tbsp lemon juice
1 clove garlic, minced
1 ½ tsp apple cider vinegar
3 tbsp water, or as needed to thin

## METHOD

To make the tahini dressing, whisk together tahini, lemon juice, garlic, apple cider vinegar, water, salt and pepper in a small bowl until smooth and creamy. Adjust water as needed to reach the desired consistency. Set aside.

In a large serving bowl, combine the quinoa, kale, chickpeas, blueberries, almonds, feta and pomegranate seeds.

Drizzle with extra virgin olive oil, season to taste and toss to combine. Pour 2 tablespoons of the tahini dressing over the bowl and gently mix everything together. Serve immediately or refrigerate for up to one day for flavours to meld.

# OMEGA-RICH MACKEREL NIÇOISE SALAD

This Mediterranean-inspired salad is like a love letter to your neurons. Mackerel delivers the omega-3s your brain craves for optimal neurotransmitter production and mental clarity. Eggs are packed with choline, important for memory and brain development. The crisp green beans provide folate and magnesium to help maintain a calm vagal tone, while olives and capers add healthy monounsaturated fats. The bright parsley is loaded with vitamin K for cognitive function.

**Serves 2**

### INGREDIENTS

- 2 mackerel fillets (grilled or canned in olive oil)
- 2 eggs
- ⅔ cup green beans
- Handful of cos (romaine) lettuce
- ½ cup chopped cucumber
- 2 tbsp roughly chopped olives
- 1 tsp roughly chopped capers
- 1 tbsp chopped fresh parsley
- ¼ cup extra virgin olive oil
- 1 tsp Dijon mustard
- Squeeze of fresh lemon juice, plus extra to serve (optional)

### METHOD

If using fresh mackerel, grill the fillets on medium heat for 3–4 minutes per side until golden and cooked through. If using canned mackerel, drain the excess oil and break into bite-sized pieces.

Boil the eggs for 7–8 minutes, then transfer to cold water to stop cooking. Peel and slice into rounds. Steam the green beans for 3-4 minutes until tender but still crisp. Rinse under cold water to maintain their bright colour.

In a serving bowl, arrange the cos lettuce, mackerel, sliced egg, green beans, cucumber, olives and capers. Sprinkle with fresh parsley.

In a small bowl, whisk together the olive oil, Dijon mustard and lemon juice to make the dressing. Drizzle the dressing over the salad and toss lightly to combine.

Serve immediately with an extra squeeze of lemon juice (if using).

# SUPER-FAST GUT-HEALING VEGETABLE SOUP

This is one of my favourite nourishing soups with gut-friendly ingredients like turmeric, garlic and fibre-rich vegetables to support digestion and immune function. Peas provide extra protein and prebiotic fibre, while warming spices enhance the flavour and boost the anti-inflammatory properties.

***Cooking tip:*** *Let the soup simmer for an extra 10 minutes to deepen the flavours. If chickpeas (garbanzo beans) cause bloating, leave them out until your gut is healed.*

**Serves 2**

## INGREDIENTS

1 tbsp extra virgin olive oil

1 clove garlic, minced

1 tsp ground turmeric

½ tsp ground coriander

½ tsp ground cumin

¼ tsp smoked paprika

½ cup chopped carrots

½ cup diced zucchini (courgette)

½ cup chopped green beans

½ cup peas

2 cups vegetable stock (broth)

Sea salt and freshly ground black pepper

### *CRISPY CHICKPEAS*

1 can chickpeas (garbanzo beans), drained and patted dry

1 tbsp extra virgin olive oil

1 tsp paprika

½ tsp cumin

Pinch of sea salt

Fresh herbs, to garnish (optional)

## METHOD

Preheat the oven to 205°C (480°F).

Heat the olive oil in a pot over medium heat. Add the garlic and sauté for 1 minute until fragrant. Stir in the turmeric, coriander, cumin and paprika, cooking for another 30 seconds to release their aromas.

Add the carrots, zucchini, green beans and peas, stirring well to coat them in the spices. Cook for 5 minutes.

Pour in the stock, bring to a simmer and let cook for 20 minutes, stirring occasionally.

Meanwhile, toss the chickpeas with oil and sprinkle with spices. Place on a baking sheet and roast in the oven for 15–20 minutes until crispy.

Taste and adjust seasoning of soup with salt and pepper as needed.

Serve warm, garnished with crispy chickpeas and fresh herbs such as parsley or coriander (if using).

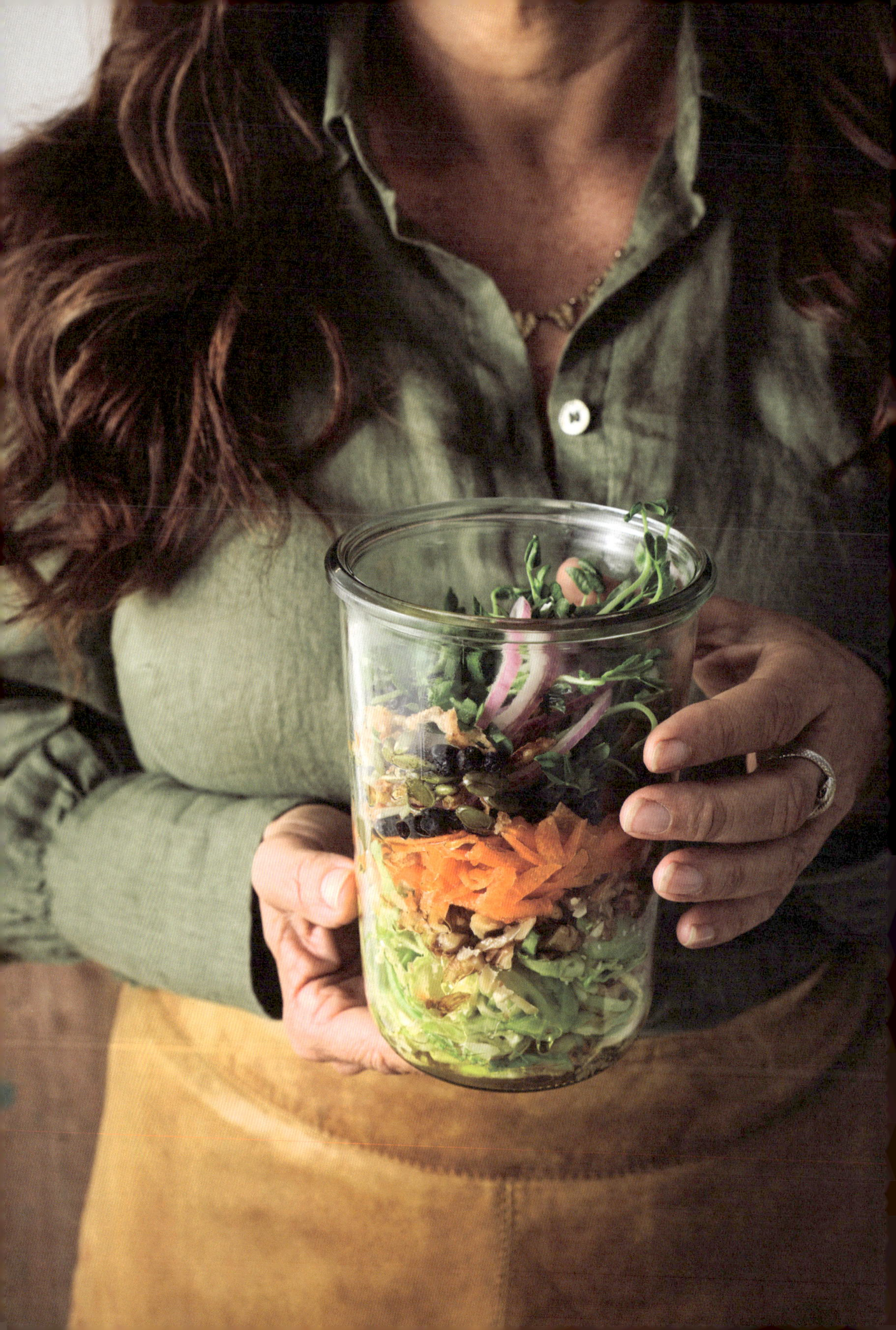

# MASON JAR BRUSSELS & WALNUT LAYERED SALAD

This vibrant layered salad is your body's fire extinguisher, packed with potent anti-inflammatory warriors. The brussels sprouts are loaded with sulforaphane, a compound that activates your body's own anti-inflammatory pathways and helps neutralise harmful free radicals. Those crunchy walnuts deliver alpha-linolenic acid, an omega-3 that directly combats inflammation at the cellular level, while the ruby-red pomegranate seeds burst with anthocyanins and ellagic acid – polyphenols that act like tiny firefighters dousing inflammatory flames throughout your body. The fresh coriander and parsley are packed with antioxidants and natural compounds that support your liver's detoxification processes. Dried blueberries provide a sweet hit of pterostilbene, a powerful anti-inflammatory compound, and the pumpkin seeds contribute zinc and vitamin E to further strengthen your body's defence systems.

**Serves 1**

## INGREDIENTS

½ cup shredded brussels sprouts
¼ cup chopped walnuts
½ cup grated carrot
¼ cup pomegranate seeds
2 tbsp dried blueberries
2 tbsp microgreens or sprouts
¼ cup thinly sliced red onion
2 tbsp crispy shallots
1 tbsp pumpkin seeds (pepitas)
1 tbsp apple cider vinegar
1 tbsp extra virgin olive oil
Sea salt and freshly ground black pepper
1 tbsp chopped fresh coriander (cilantro)
1 tbsp chopped fresh parsley

## METHOD

Layer all the ingredients in a mason jar, starting with the brussels sprouts then the walnuts, carrot, pomegranate seeds, dried blueberries and microgreens.

Add thinly sliced red onion, crispy shallots and pumpkin seeds for extra texture. Drizzle with apple cider vinegar and olive oil. Season with salt and pepper. Sprinkle with fresh coriander and parsley.

Close the jar and shake well before eating to distribute the dressing and flavours.

# BLACK BEAN TACO BOWL WITH TAHINI DRESSING

Your mitochondria are about to go into overdrive with this rainbow-powered energy bowl that's practically bursting with cellular fuel. The protein-packed black beans and quinoa team up to deliver sustained energy. Vibrant purple cabbage shreds are loaded with anthocyanins that protect your mitochondria from energy-sapping oxidative stress, while the roasted sweet potato cubes provide beta-carotene and natural sugars for quick cellular uptake. The creamy tahini dressing delivers a hefty dose of magnesium. Crispy spiced chickpeas (garbanzo beans) bring additional protein and B vitamins, while the iron-rich spinach helps optimise oxygen delivery to your hardworking cells.

**Serves 2–3**

### INGREDIENTS

*FOR ROASTING*

1 medium sweet potato, cubed

1 tsp extra virgin olive oil

Sea salt

½ cup chickpeas (garbanzo beans), drained and patted dry thoroughly

½ tsp ground cumin

½ tsp garlic powder

½ tsp onion powder

½ tsp smoked paprika

Pinch of ground chilli, to taste

*FOR THE BOWL*

½ cup quinoa, cooked

½ cup black beans

½ red onion, chopped

½ cup baby spinach

¼ purple cabbage, shredded

½ avocado, sliced

½ cup crumbled feta or goat's cheese

2 tbsp pumpkin seeds (pepitas)

Microgreens, to garnish

*FOR THE TAHINI DRESSING*

2 tbsp tahini

1 tbsp lemon juice

1 small garlic clove, minced

1 tsp maple syrup

¼ tsp ground cumin

Sea salt and freshly ground black pepper

Water to thin

*OPTIONAL TOPPINGS*

Fresh coriander (cilantro) leaves

Lemon wedges

Lemon zest

Tortilla chips

## METHOD

Preheat the oven to 200°C (400°F). Line a baking tray with baking (parchment) paper.

On one side of the tray, toss the sweet potato cubes with a little olive oil and salt. On the other side, toss chickpeas with cumin, garlic and onion powders, smoked paprika, chilli, the remaining olive oil and salt. Roast for 20–25 minutes, tossing halfway through. The chickpeas should be crispy and the sweet potatoes tender.

Meanwhile, prepare the tahini dressing. In a small bowl, whisk together the tahini, lemon juice, garlic, maple syrup, cumin, salt and pepper. Add water gradually until you reach your desired consistency.

To assemble the taco bowl, layer the cooked quinoa and black beans as the base. Add the red onion, roasted sweet potatoes, baby spinach, purple cabbage, avocado slices and feta or goat's cheese. Top with the roasted chickpeas, pumpkin seeds and microgreens.

Drizzle with the tahini dressing and garnish with fresh coriander, lemon wedges, lemon zest and feta (if using). Add some tortilla chips too if you like a little extra crunch.

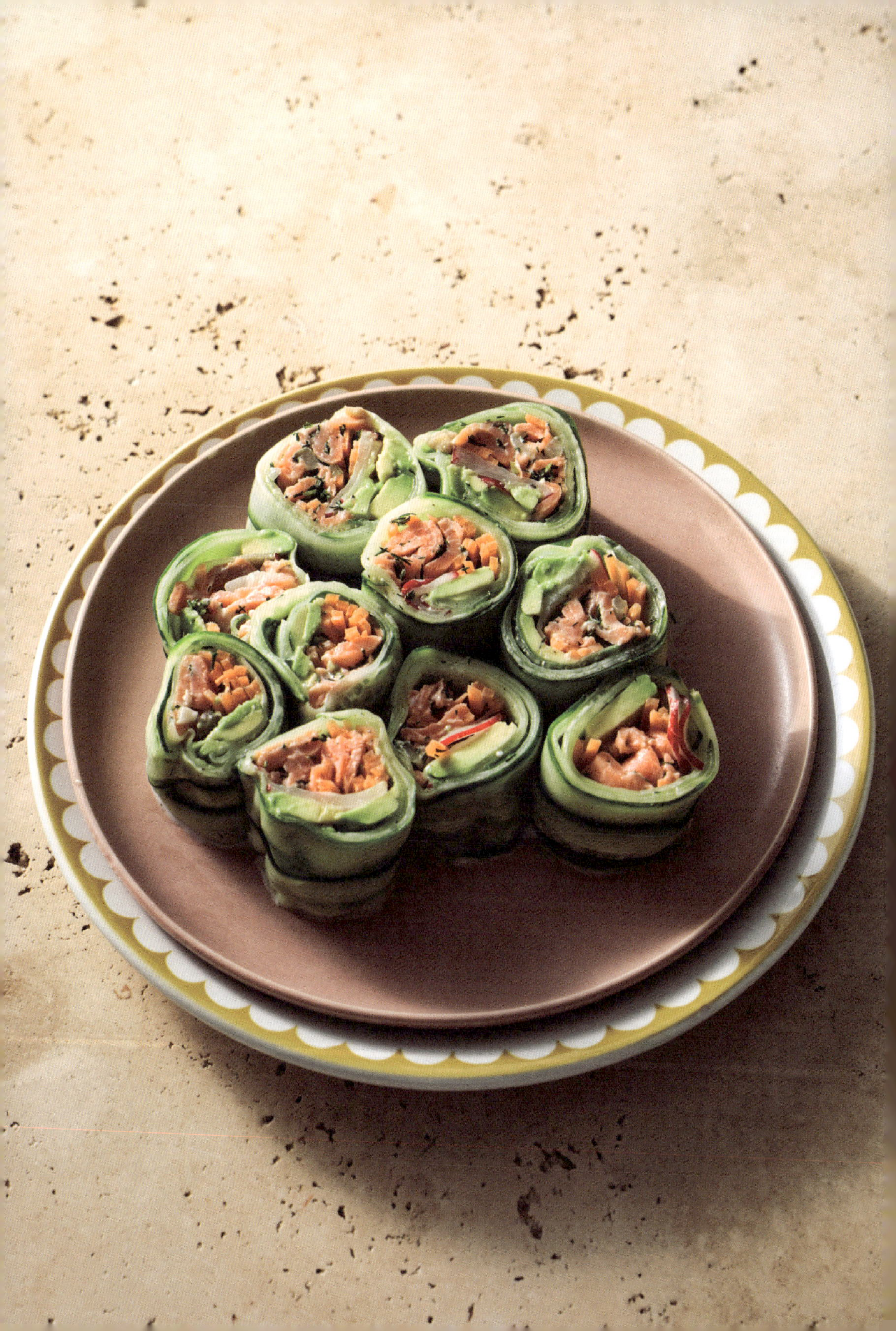

# CUCUMBER ROLLS WITH SMOKED TROUT

Designed to nourish your brain and calm your nervous system, these elegant grain-free rolls actively support your mental clarity, reduce inflammation and help your nervous system find its natural calm. The omega-3-rich smoked trout delivers concentrated DHA and EPA. The creamy tzatziki is packed with probiotics that support your gut–brain axis. Fresh dill provides folate and antioxidants that support healthy neurotransmitter production. The silky avocado slices contribute healthy monounsaturated fats that help your body absorb all those brain-boosting nutrients, while the crisp carrots and radishes add B vitamins.

**Serves 2**

## INGREDIENTS

- 2 long continental (English) cucumbers (choose a firm, wide one for best results)
- 100 g (3½ oz) smoked trout fillet, flaked
- 2 tbsp tzatziki
- Sprigs of fresh dill, finely chopped
- ¼ lemon, juiced
- Sea salt and freshly ground black pepper
- 1 small carrot, julienned
- 3 radishes, finely sliced
- ½ avocado, thinly sliced
- Pinch of sesame seeds, to serve (optional)

## METHOD

Use a vegetable peeler or mandolin to shave the cucumbers lengthways into long, wide ribbons. You'll need about 20 ribbons for two servings. Choose cucumbers that are straight and wide for easier rolling. If the slices seem too thin or delicate, layer two ribbons together, slightly overlapping to reinforce them. Pat the slices dry with a paper towel (kitchen paper) to prevent sogginess.

In a bowl, mix the flaked smoked trout with the tzatziki, chopped dill, lemon juice, and a pinch of salt and pepper.

On a large piece of cling (plastic) wrap, arrange half the cucumber slices vertically side by side and overlapping slightly to create one large square of cucumber slices. Pat dry with paper towel.

On the vertical edge, layer half the avocado, radish, carrot and smoked trout mixture.

Use the cling wrap to roll up tightly, pulling the wrap off as you go. Cut the roll crosswise into six pieces. Repeat with the remaining cucumber and fillings and serve with sesame seeds (if using).

---

*SERVING SUGGESTION*

Plate with a drizzle of olive oil, a few extra dill sprigs, and a sprinkle of black or white sesame seeds for added fibre and flavour.

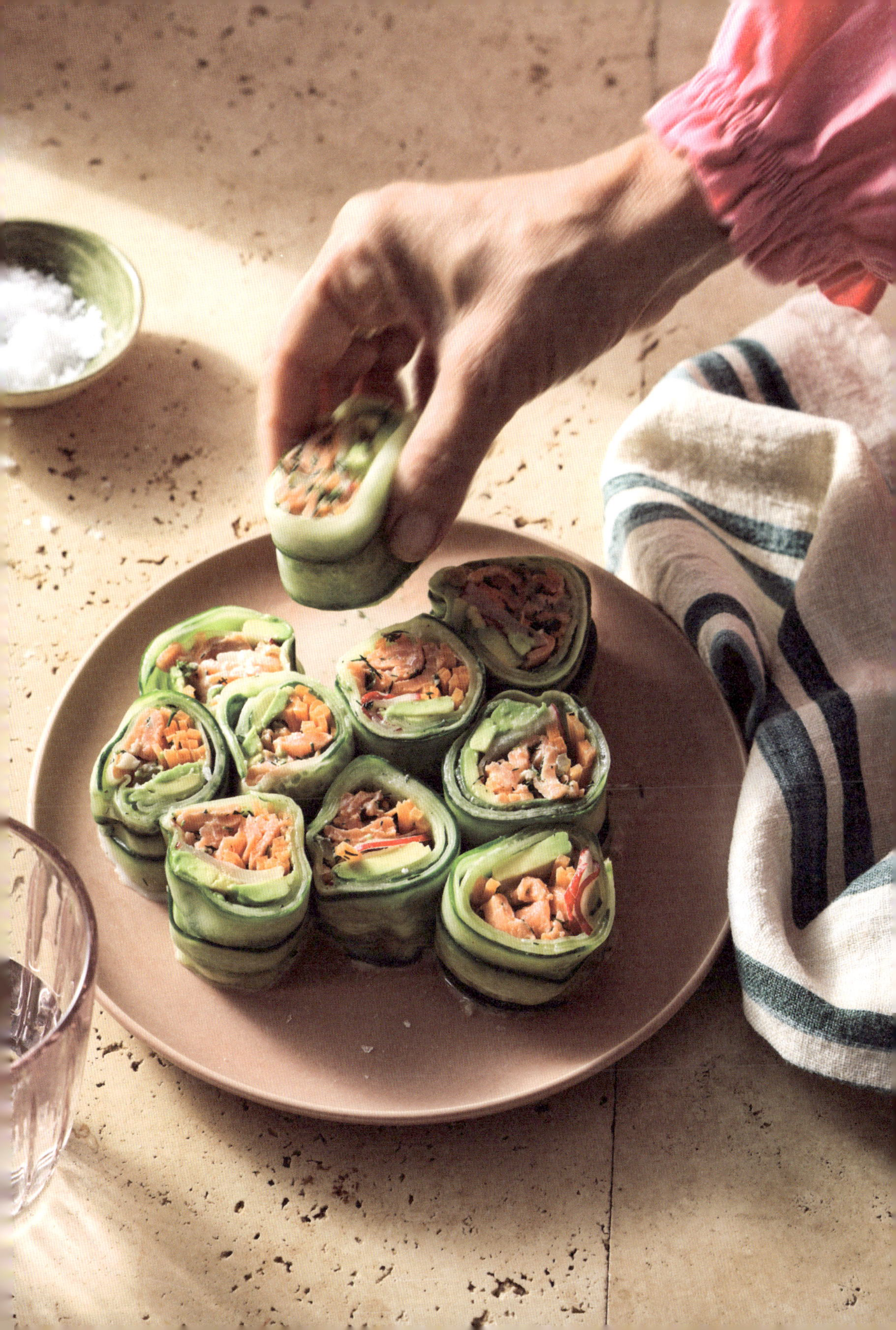

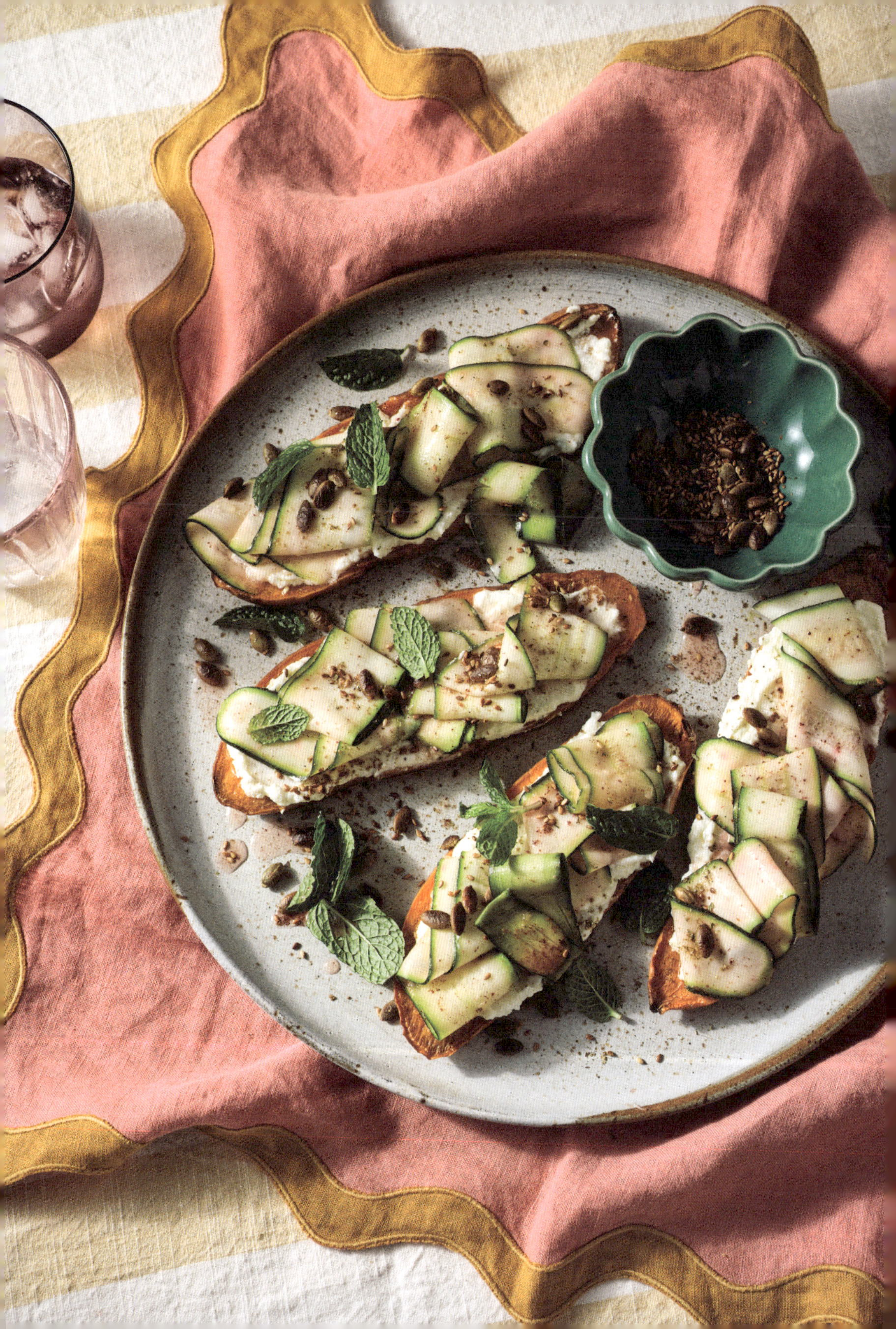

# SWEET POTATO 'TOAST' WITH LABNEH & ZA'ATAR

A MAP-friendly alternative to toast, these sweet potato slices are slow-roasted for better digestion and topped with creamy labneh, which is probiotic-rich and soothing for the gut. Zucchini (courgette) ribbons are lightly marinated and finished with anti-inflammatory za'atar-spiced seeds.

**Serves 2**

## INGREDIENTS

1 large sweet potato, cut lengthways into 1 cm (½ inch) slices

1 tbsp extra virgin olive oil

Sea salt

1 zucchini (courgette), shaved into ribbons

Juice of ½ lemon

½ tsp sumac

1 tbsp mixed seeds (sunflower, pumpkin/pepitas, sesame)

1 tsp za'atar

Fresh mint leaves, to serve

100 g (3½ oz) labneh

## METHOD

Preheat oven to 180°C (350°F). Brush the sweet potato slices with olive oil and a pinch of salt, then bake for 25–30 minutes until golden and tender.

In a bowl, toss zucchini ribbons with lemon juice and sumac. Leave to marinate for at least 10 minutes.

Lightly toast seeds in a dry pan for 2–3 minutes, then stir through the za'atar.

Spread the labneh over the baked sweet potato slices. Top with marinated zucchini and scatter with za'atar-spiced seeds and mint leaves.

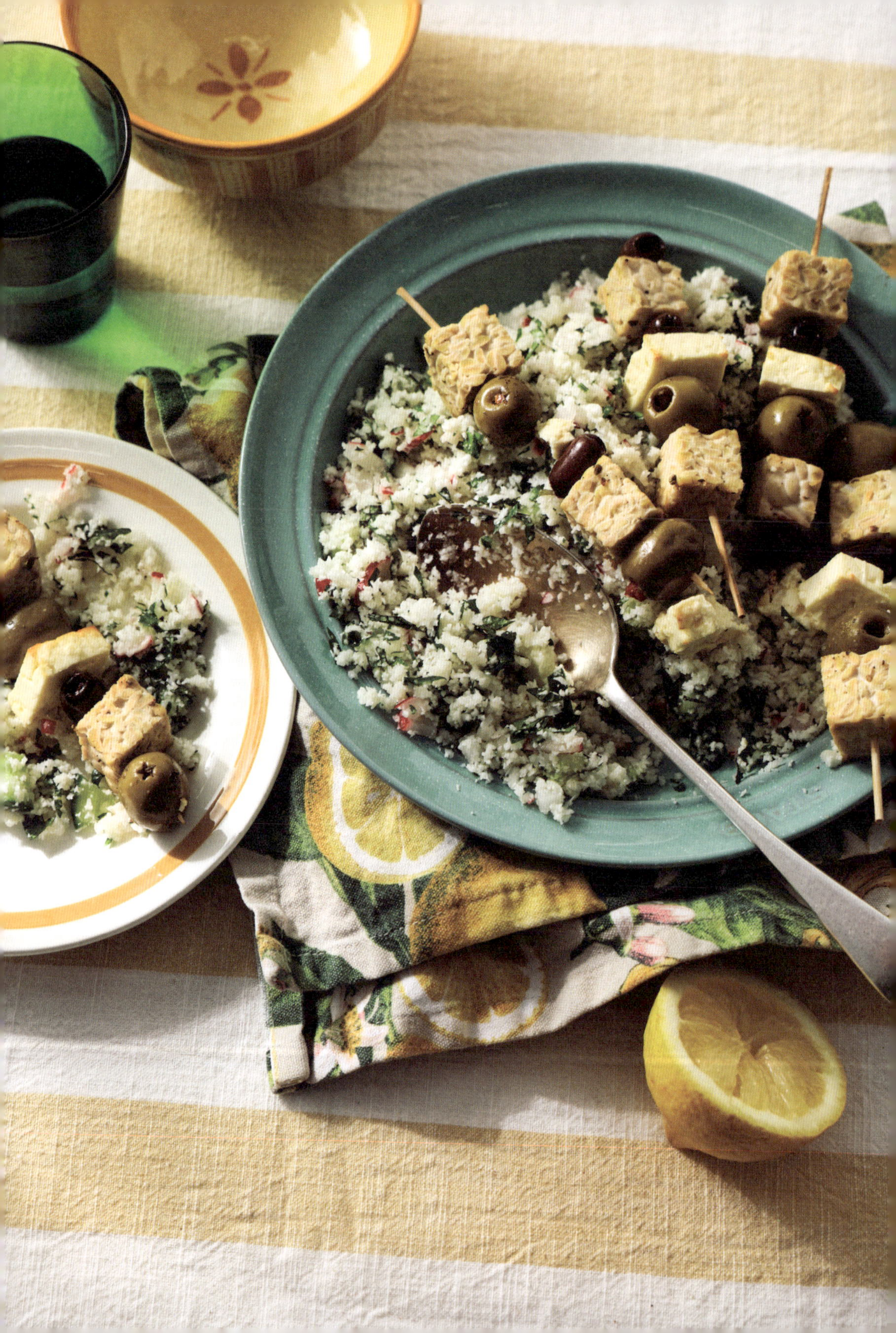

# TEMPEH, OLIVE & FETA SKEWERS

Your mitochondria are about to get a Mediterranean makeover with these vibrant skewers that pack serious cellular fuel into every bite. The fermented tempeh is loaded with protein, probiotics and B vitamins that support energy metabolism, while those briny olives provide healthy monounsaturated fats. The tangy feta adds quality protein and calcium for muscle function, and when air-fried, everything gets a gorgeous golden caramelisation without the inflammatory damage of high-heat cooking. But here's where it gets clever: that herb-packed cauliflower tabbouleh isn't just a grain-free twist – it's bursting with vitamin C from the fresh parsley and mint, while the sulforaphane in cauliflower helps your cells' natural detox processes run smoothly.

**Serves 2**

## INGREDIENTS

*SKEWERS*

200 g (7 oz) tempeh, cut into cubes

1 tbsp extra virgin olive oil

1 tsp dried oregano

Juice of ½ lemon

Sea salt and freshly ground black pepper

8–10 mixed olives (green or black), pitted

80 g (2¾ oz) feta, cut into cubes (Greek feta is more authentic but Danish holds its form better)

4–6 bamboo or metal skewers

*CAULIFLOWER TABBOULEH*

½ head cauliflower, grated or pulsed into rice-sized grains

½ cucumber, finely diced

6 cherry-sized radishes, finely chopped

Small bunch fresh parsley, finely chopped

2 tbsp finely chopped fresh mint

Juice of 1 lemon

2 tbsp extra virgin olive oil, plus extra to garnish

Sea salt

Fresh mint leaves, to garnish

## METHOD

Place the tempeh cubes in a bowl with olive oil, lemon juice, oregano, and a pinch of salt and pepper. Toss gently to coat and marinate for at least 20 minutes, or longer in the fridge to deepen the flavour.

To make the tabbouleh, place the riced cauliflower in a bowl, sprinkle with ½ teaspoon sea salt and let sit for 15–20 minutes. Squeeze out any water that has been released before adding the remaining ingredients. This softens the cauliflower and mellows its flavour. Add the cucumber, radishes, parsley and mint. Dress with lemon juice, olive oil and salt. Mix well and let sit for the flavours to meld.

To make the skewers, thread the tempeh, olives and feta alternately onto the skewers. Handle the feta gently to avoid crumbling. Double up any small olives if needed for balance.

Air-fry the skewers at 180°C (350°F) for 8–10 minutes, turning halfway, until the tempeh is golden and feta is slightly crisp.

Serve the skewers over the cauliflower tabbouleh. Drizzle with extra olive oil and garnish with a few fresh mint leaves.

### *SERVING TIPS*

Served cold, these skewers are perfect for packed lunches or mezze platters. Add a sprinkle of hemp seeds or crushed pumpkin seeds (pepitas) for extra texture and anti-inflammatory benefits.

Using Greek feta will give the most authentic Mediterranean flavour. But the firm, creamy structure of Danish feta will work better on the skewers.

# GRILLED STONE FRUIT SALAD WITH ENDIVE

This vibrant salad layers smoky grilled stone fruit with peppery greens, umami-rich parmesan and fresh herbs for a refreshing anti-inflammatory lunch. The ginger-citrus dressing brings digestive support and a gentle heat, while toasted macadamias add crunch, healthy fats and a subtle garlic aroma. The antioxidant-rich stone fruits, omega-7 fatty acids from macadamias and polyphenol-packed bitter greens work together to actively combat inflammatory pathways throughout your body. This dish captures the essence of a modern Mediterranean plate – colourful, aromatic and deeply nourishing.

**Serves 2**

## INGREDIENTS

*SALAD*

2 ripe nectarine or peach, halved and pitted

1 tsp extra virgin olive oil

1 head endive, leaves separated

1 large handful of rocket (arugula)

4–6 fresh basil leaves, torn

2 tbsp fresh mint leaves, torn

20 g (¾ oz) parmesan, shaved

*CRUSHED MACADAMIAS*

40 g (1½ oz) raw macadamias

1 tsp extra virgin olive oil

1 small garlic clove, finely grated

*DRESSING*

1 tsp grated fresh ginger

Juice of 1 lime

Juice of ½ orange

½ small green chilli, deseeded and finely chopped

2 tbsp extra virgin olive oil

Sea salt

## METHOD

To make the dressing, whisk together the grated ginger, lime juice, orange juice, chilli and olive oil in a small bowl. Season with salt to taste. Set aside to let flavours develop.

To make the crushed macadamias, roughly chop the nuts. Heat the olive oil in a small pan over medium–low heat. Add the garlic and nuts, and toast gently for 2–3 minutes until fragrant and golden, stirring often. Set aside to cool slightly.

To make the salad, brush the cut sides of the stone fruit with a touch of olive oil. Grill on a hot chargrill pan or barbecue (grill) for 2–3 minutes per side until charred marks appear and the fruit is slightly softened. Remove and slice thickly.

On a large serving plate or two individual plates, layer endive leaves, rocket, basil and mint. Arrange the sliced grilled fruit on top. Drizzle with the ginger-citrus dressing and scatter over the shaved parmesan and toasted garlic macadamias.

### *SERVING TIP*

For an added protein boost, pair this salad with grilled tempeh or cold poached white fish. Serve immediately while the fruit is still warm for a contrast in texture and temperature.

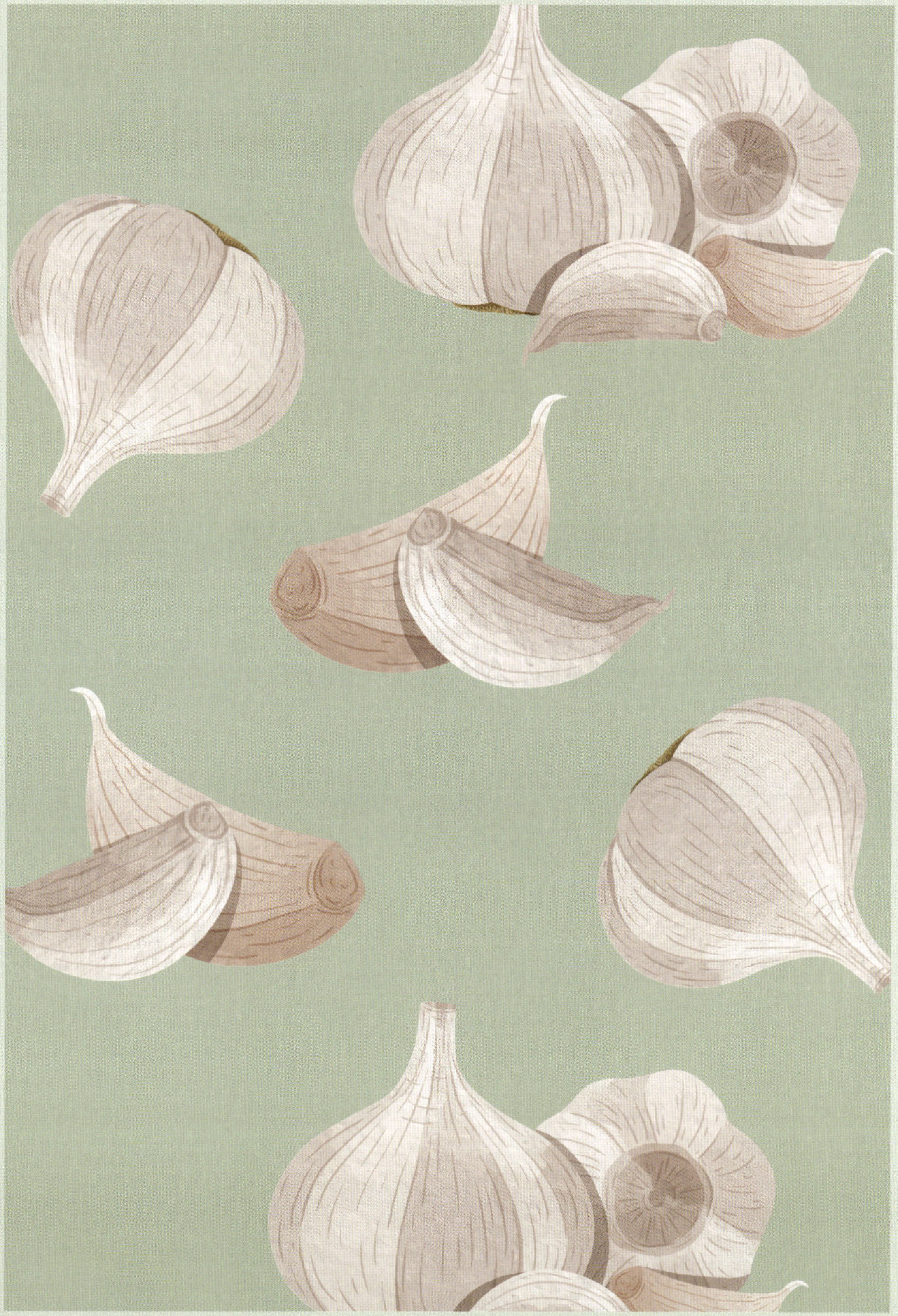

# SLOW-ROASTED ARTICHOKE HEARTS WITH LEMON-CAPER-AVOCADO WHIP

This vibrant, texture-rich dish layers MAP ingredients into a nourishing salad that's both soothing and invigorating. The slow-roasted artichokes are gently spiced to elevate their anti-inflammatory potential. Paired with creamy lemon-caper-avocado whip and crunchy smashed cucumber, this meal has gut-supportive prebiotics, antioxidants and healthy fats. But here's the cellular energy magic: artichokes are packed with magnesium and potassium – essential minerals your mitochondria need for efficient ATP production – while their unique prebiotic fibres feed beneficial gut bacteria that support energy metabolism. Your metabolism will be kept humming smoothly all day long.

**Serves 2**

## INGREDIENTS

*ROASTED ARTICHOKES*

1 jar (approx. 200 g/7 oz drained) artichoke hearts in water or brine (not oil-packed)

1 tbsp extra virgin olive oil

1 garlic clove, finely minced

Zest of ½ lemon

1 tsp Healing herb & spice blend (page 245)

Pinch of sea salt and freshly ground black pepper

*SMASHED CUCUMBER*

½ large cucumber

Sea salt

1 tsp apple cider vinegar

*LEMON-CAPER-AVOCADO WHIP*

1 ripe avocado

Juice of ½ lemon

1 tbsp capers, rinsed and chopped

1 tbsp Greek yogurt

1 tbsp extra virgin olive oil

Sea salt and freshly ground black pepper

*HERB SALAD*

1 handful mixed salad leaves (e.g. rocket/arugula, endive, baby spinach)

1 tbsp roughly chopped fresh parsley

1 tbsp fresh mint leaves, torn

1 tsp chopped fresh dill

*DRESSING*

Juice of ½ lemon

1 tbsp extra virgin olive oil

Sea salt

### METHOD

Preheat the oven to 160°C (315°F). Line a baking tray with baking (parchment) paper.

To make the dressing, whisk together the lemon juice, olive oil and sea salt.

Drain the artichoke hearts and gently pat dry. Toss with the olive oil, garlic, lemon zest, spice blend, and salt and pepper to taste until evenly coated. Arrange on the lined baking tray and roast for 35–40 minutes, turning once, until golden and lightly crisped on the edges.

To make the smashed cucumber, lightly smash the cucumber with the flat of a knife or rolling pin, then roughly chop. Sprinkle with the sea salt and apple cider vinegar and set aside to marinate.

To make the lemon-caper-avocado whip, put all the ingredients in a blender and blend until creamy.

To make the salad, combine the mixed salad leaves with parsley, mint and dill. Toss through the dressing.

To assemble, spread the lemon-caper-avocado whip across the base of each serving plate. Top with smashed cucumber then warm roasted artichokes. Finish with the herb salad and an extra drizzle of dressing.

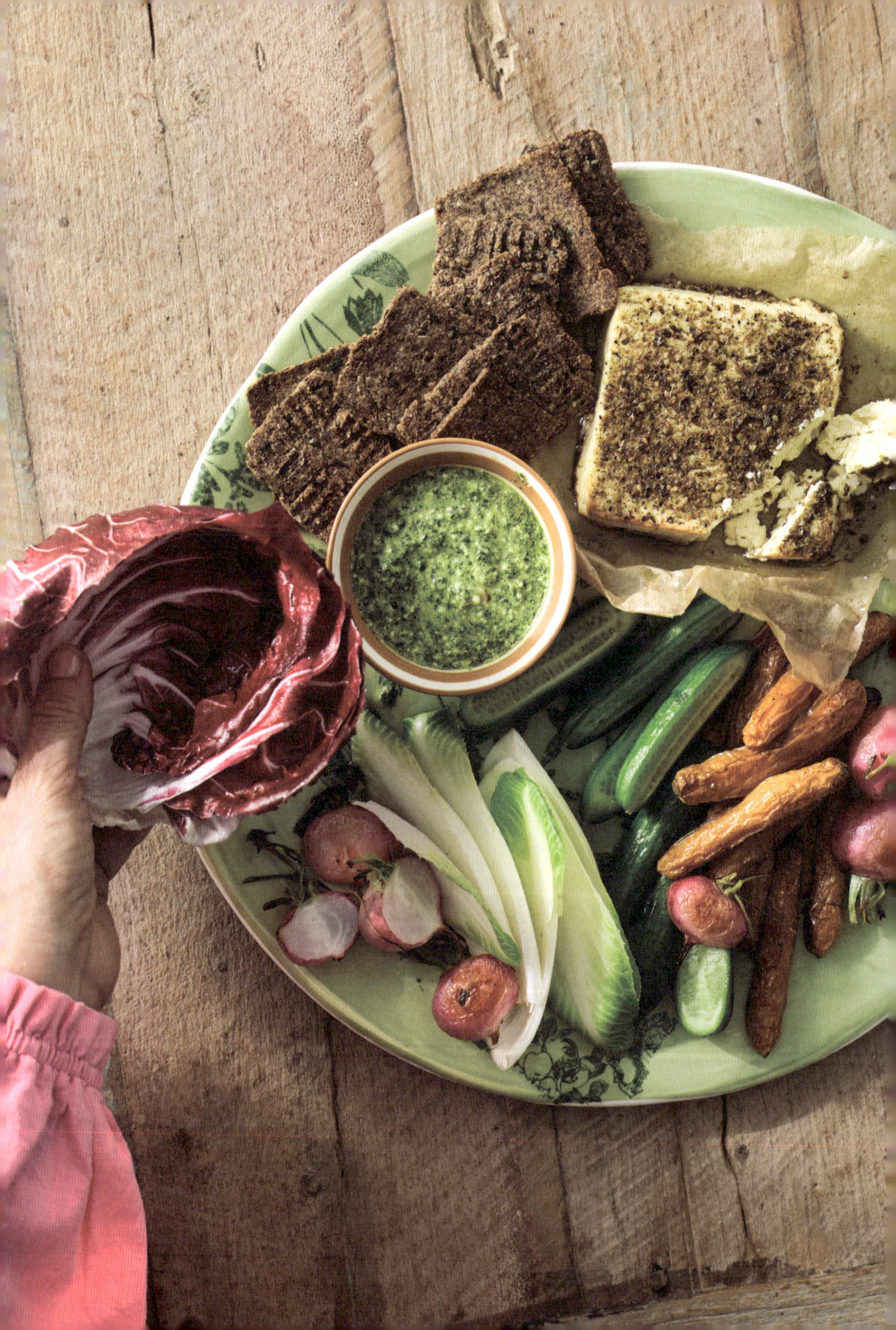

# MEDITERRANEAN MEZZE PLATTER

This colourful mezze platter is a MAP-style celebration of anti-inflammatory abundance. Featuring roasted feta for creamy richness, crisp and roasted crudités, sardine crackers, and a vibrant herb pesto packed with phytonutrients, it's a feast for the senses and a gift for the gut. Every bite delivers prebiotic fibre, healthy fats and inflammation-soothing compounds, helping to calm the nervous system and energise your cells.

**Serves 2–4 (as a light lunch or sharing plate)**

## INGREDIENTS

*ROASTED FETA*

200 g (7 oz) feta (preferably sheep's milk)

1 tbsp extra virgin olive oil

½ tsp dried oregano

½ tsp za'atar

Freshly ground black pepper

*CRUDITÉS*

4 baby cucumbers, halved lengthways

6–8 whole baby carrots, scrubbed

6 radishes, halved

1 small head radicchio, leaves separated

1 small endive, leaves separated

1 tsp extra virgin olive oil (for roasting carrots and radishes)

Pinch of sea salt

*HERB PESTO DIP*

½ cup fresh basil leaves

½ cup fresh mint leaves

¼ cup fresh parsley leaves

2 tbsp walnuts or pine nuts

1 tbsp nutritional yeast or grated parmesan (optional)

1 small garlic clove

Juice of ½ lemon

4 tbsp extra virgin olive oil

Sea salt and freshly ground black pepper

Splash of water to thin, if needed

4–6 Sardine crackers, to serve (page 230)

Extra olive oil and sumac, to garnish

### METHOD

Preheat the oven to 180°C (350ºF).

Place the feta in a small baking dish. Drizzle with olive oil, sprinkle with oregano, za'atar and pepper. Roast for 20–25 minutes until golden and softened.

On a separate tray, toss the baby carrots and radishes with olive oil and sea salt. Roast for 15–20 minutes until just tender and lightly caramelised.

Meanwhile, prepare the pesto. Combine the basil, mint, parsley, walnuts, nutritional yeast, garlic, lemon juice and olive oil in a food processor. Blitz until smooth, adding a splash of water to thin as needed. Season with salt and pepper to taste.

To arrange the mezze platter, place the roasted feta in the centre, surrounded by the roasted radishes and carrots; fresh cucumber halves, radicchio and endive; and sardine crackers. Serve with a generous bowl of the herb pesto for dipping, and a drizzle of olive oil and sprinkle of sumac.

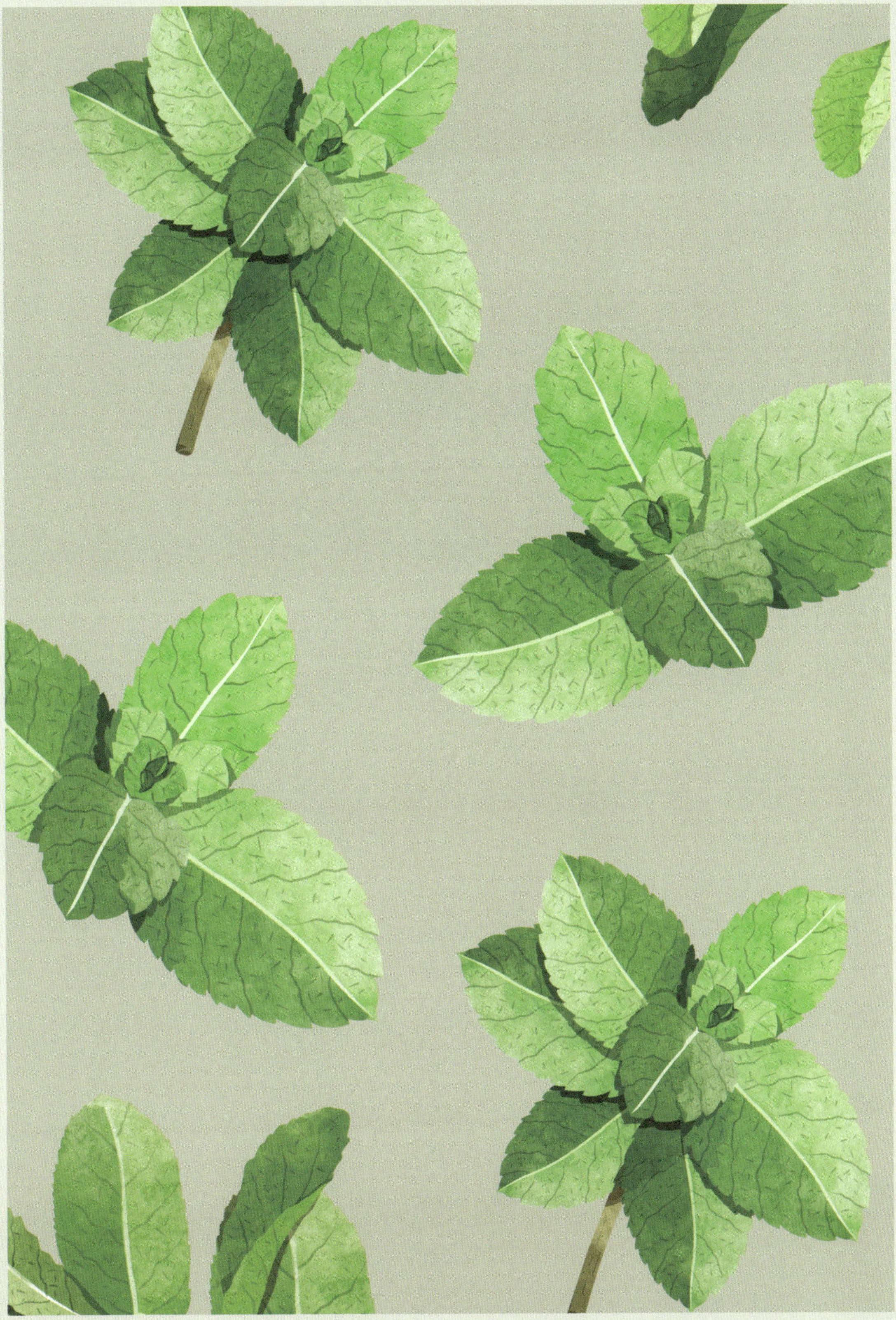

# DINNERS

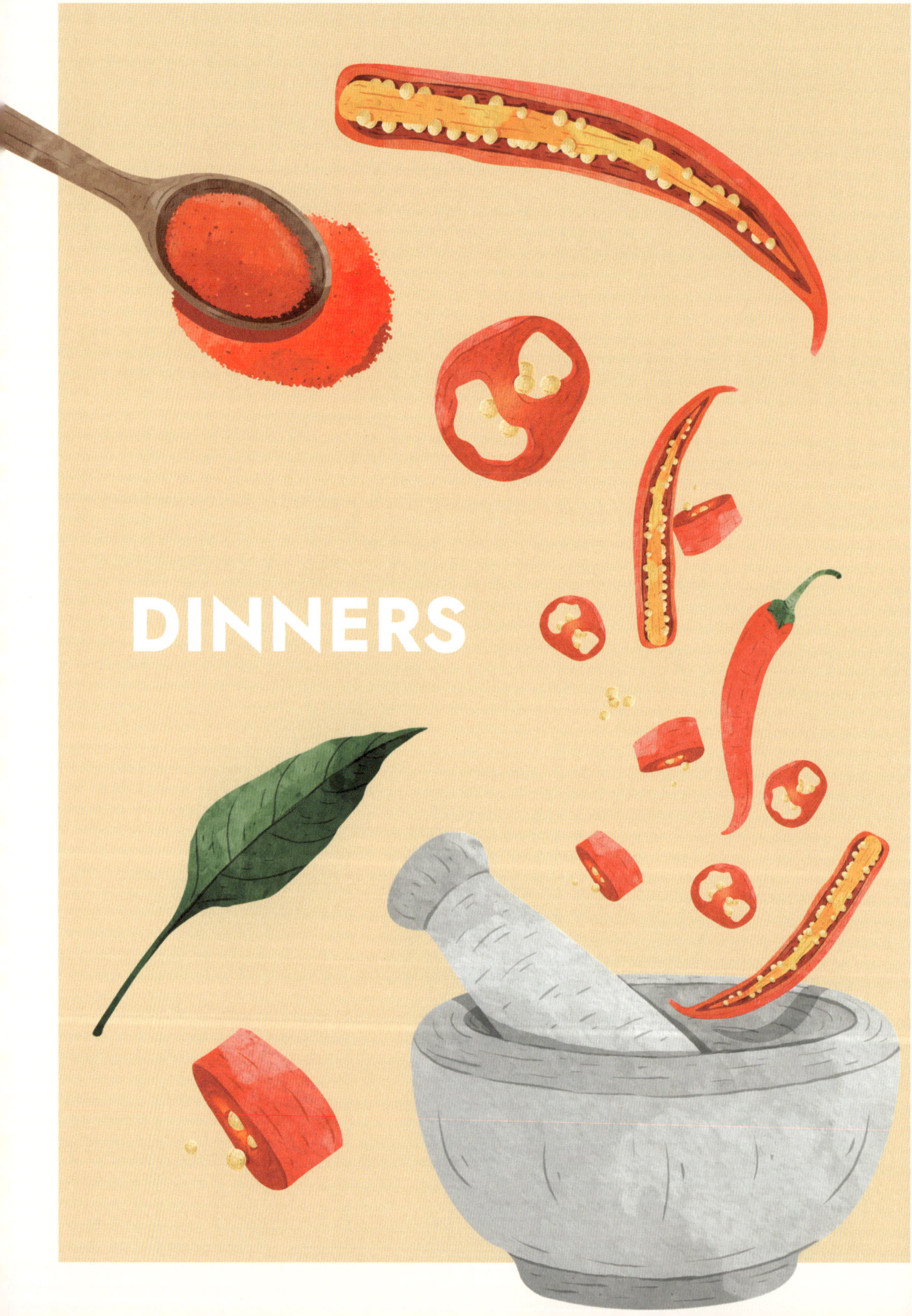

# LEE'S FISH PIE WITH CAULIFLOWER MASH

**Serves 4–6**

## INGREDIENTS

*FISH FILLING*

1 tbsp extra virgin olive oil

½ onion, diced

1 celery stalk, diced

2 cloves garlic, minced

½ tsp curry powder

1 litre (1 quart) chicken stock

2 turnips, peeled and cut into 2.5 cm (1 inch) cubes

1 tsp dried (or fresh) tarragon, chopped

4 fillets white fish (barramundi, flathead, snapper), skin and bones removed, cut into chunks

1 cup peas (fresh or frozen)

2 eggs, hard-boiled and chopped

1 cup additive-free coconut milk

Sea salt and freshly ground black pepper

*CAULIFLOWER MASH*

1 head cauliflower, chopped into florets

¼ cup nutritional yeast

1 tbsp extra virgin olive oil or ghee

Sea salt and freshly ground black pepper

Fresh flat-leaf (Italian) parsley, chopped, to garnish

## METHOD

In a large pot, heat the olive oil over medium heat. Add the onion, celery and garlic to the pot and sauté for 3–4 minutes until softened and fragrant.

Stir in the curry powder and cook for another 30 seconds to toast the spices. Add the chicken stock, turnips and dried tarragon. Bring to the boil, then reduce heat and simmer for 15–20 minutes until the turnips are tender.

Add the fish chunks, peas and coconut milk. Simmer for another 5–7 minutes until the fish is cooked through and the mixture has thickened. (Check with a fork to see if it flakes easily.)

Gently fold in the chopped hard-boiled eggs and season with salt and pepper to taste. Set aside.

While the fish filling is cooking, make the cauliflower mash. Bring a large pot of salted water to the boil. Add the cauliflower florets and cook for 8–10 minutes until fork-tender.

Drain the cauliflower and transfer it to a food processor or large bowl. Add the nutritional yeast, olive oil, and salt and pepper to taste. Blend until smooth and creamy. You can add a little water or more oil as needed to achieve the desired consistency.

To make the pie, preheat your oven to 180°C (350°F).

Transfer the fish filling mixture into a baking dish, spreading it evenly. Carefully spoon the cauliflower mash on top of the fish filling, spreading it out with a spatula to cover the entire surface.

Use a fork to gently score the top of the mash, creating a crisscross pattern. This will give it a nice texture when baked. Place the baking dish in the oven and bake for 20–25 minutes, or until the top of the mash is lightly golden.

When ready, remove from the oven and garnish with fresh flat-leaf parsley.

# TURMERIC-SPICED CHICKEN WITH HERB SAUCE

This succulent chicken dish is infused with warming spices and a vibrant herb sauce, featuring anti-inflammatory ingredients and bright Mediterranean flavours. Perfect for a nourishing, flavour-packed meal.

**Cooking tips**

*Bring the chicken to room temperature before roasting to ensure even cooking.*
*Halfway through cooking, use the pan juices to baste the chicken.*
*Make extra herb sauce – it's great on roasted veggies, grilled fish or as a dressing!*

**Serves 2–3**

### INGREDIENTS

4 bone-in, skin-on chicken thighs
1 red onion, cut into wedges
2 lemons, halved
3–4 fresh bay leaves
3 sprigs fresh thyme

*SPICE RUB*

1½ tsp ground turmeric
1½ tsp smoked paprika
1½ tsp ground cumin
1 tsp ground coriander
¾ tsp freshly ground black pepper
½ tsp cinnamon
3 cloves garlic, minced
1½ tbsp grated fresh ginger
Zest of 1 lemon
3 tbsp extra virgin olive oil
Sea salt

*CHERMOULA-STYLE HERB SAUCE*

¾ cup fresh parsley
½ cup fresh coriander
¼ cup fresh mint
3 cloves garlic
1 green chilli (optional)
1 preserved lemon (or juice of 1 lemon)
2 tbsp capers
⅓ cup extra virgin olive oil
1½ tsp ground cumin
¾ tsp smoked paprika
Sea salt and freshly ground black pepper

*TO SERVE*

Roasted vegetable salad (page 167) or a side of sauerkraut
¼ cup toasted pine nuts
¼ cup pomegranate seeds
Extra fresh herbs (parsley, mint, coriander)
Greek yogurt (optional)

## METHOD

To make the spice rub, in a small bowl, mix all the spice rub ingredients into a thick paste.

Pat the chicken dry and score it, then rub the spice mixture evenly over each piece. Let marinate for at least 2–4 hours, or overnight in the fridge for deeper flavour.

Preheat the oven to 200°C (400°F).

Place the chicken in a roasting pan with the red onion wedges, lemon halves, bay leaves and thyme sprigs around it. Drizzle lightly with extra olive oil. Roast for 35–40 minutes, basting with the pan juices halfway through, until the skin is crispy. Halfway through, turn the red onion and baste to collect the flavours.

Meanwhile, make the chermoula-style herb sauce. While the chicken roasts, blend or finely chop all the ingredients until slightly chunky. Adjust seasoning to taste.

When the chicken is cooked, let it rest for 5–10 minutes to retain juices.

Plate the chicken and drizzle with the herb sauce. Garnish with pine nuts, pomegranate seeds and extra herbs. Serve with roasted vegetables, pine nuts, pomegranate seeds, extra herbs and a dollop of Greek yogurt (if using).

# CAPER-CRUSTED SALMON WITH WHIPPED GREEK YOGURT

The omega-3-rich salmon delivers concentrated DHA and EPA to your brain for optimal neurotransmitter production and mental clarity. The vibrant caper and herb crust is packed with antioxidants and B vitamins that support healthy nerve function, while garlic provides compounds that help protect brain cells from oxidative stress.

**Serves 2**

## INGREDIENTS

2 salmon fillets, skin on, at room temperature
½ cup finely chopped fresh parsley
3 tbsp finely chopped capers
3 cloves garlic, minced
Juice and zest of 2 lemons
1 tbsp paprika
¼ cup panko (breadcrumbs)
¼ cup finely grated parmesan
2 tbsp Dijon mustard
½ cup Greek yogurt
Extra virgin olive oil
Sea salt and freshly ground black pepper
2 bunches asparagus, halved
Lemon slices, to serve

## METHOD

Preheat the oven to 200°C (390°F).

Line a baking tray with baking (parchment) paper. Place salmon fillets on the tray and set aside.

In a bowl, mix olive oil, parsley, capers, two of the garlic cloves, half the lemon juice and zest, and paprika. Remove 2 heaped tablespoons and set aside for serving.

Add panko and parmesan to the remaining mixture and stir well.

Spread a tablespoon of mustard to the top and sides of each salmon fillet then add an even layer of the panko mixture. Bake for 15 minutes, until firm and flaky.

Whip Greek yogurt with lemon juice and the remaining zest and garlic.

Add the asparagus to boiling water and blanch for 3–5 minutes. Drain and season with a drizzle of olive oil, lemon juice and a sprinkle of salt.

Remove salmon from the oven and serve with whipped yogurt, asparagus and a spoonful of the reserved caper mixture.

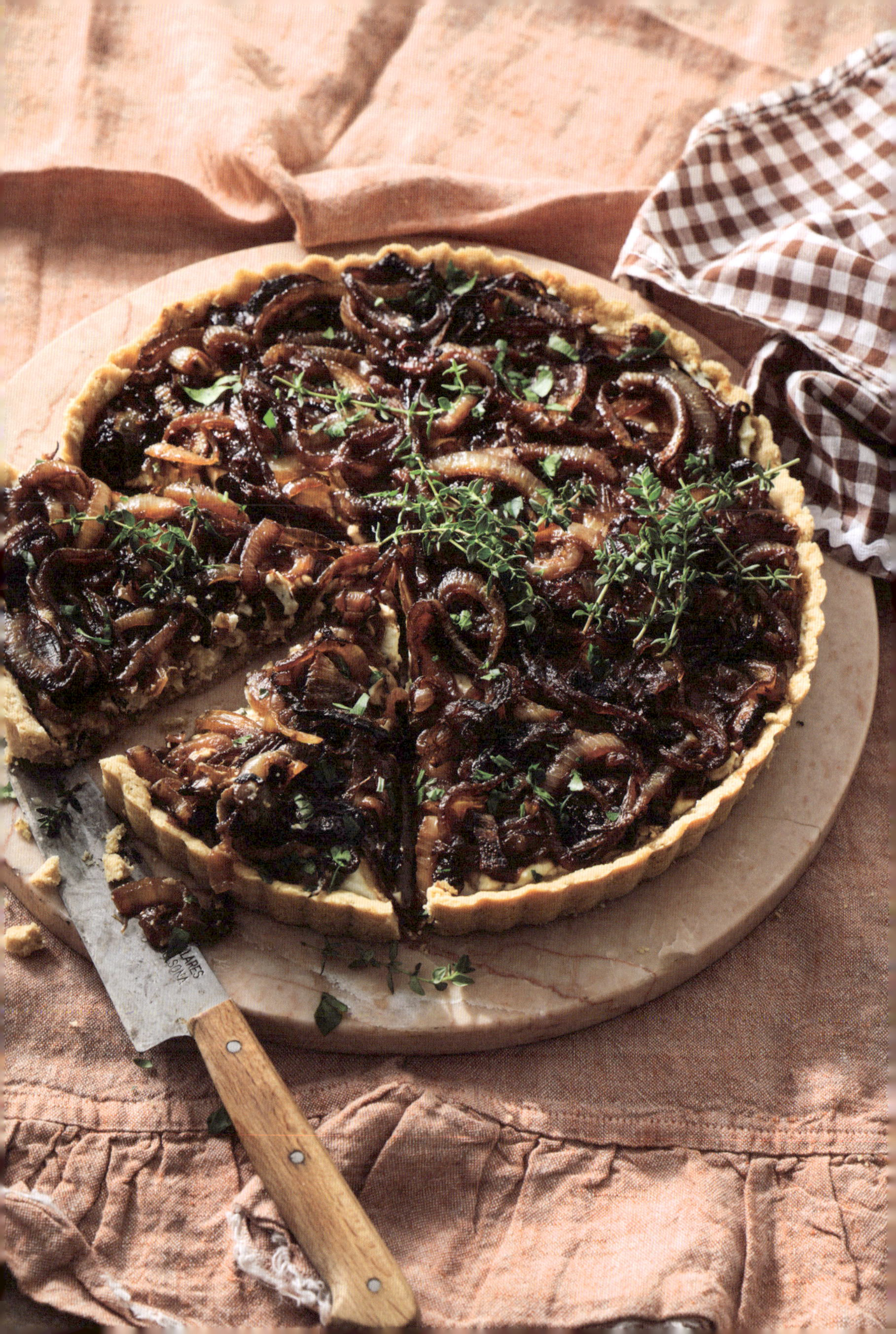

# CHEESY HERB & CARAMELISED ONION TART

This Mediterranean-inspired tart transforms simple ingredients into serious cellular fuel for your energy-hungry mitochondria. The nutrient-dense almond meal crust delivers magnesium, vitamin E and healthy fats, while those slowly caramelised onions are packed with quercetin. The creamy feta and Greek yogurt filling provides all the essential amino acids for cellular repair, plus probiotics that support your gut–brain-energy axis. And the fresh herbs deliver iron, B vitamins and antioxidants that keep your metabolic pathways running smoothly.

**Serves 4–6**

## INGREDIENTS

*TART CRUST*

200 g (7 oz) almond meal

1 tsp bicarbonate of soda (baking soda)

½ tsp sea salt

½ tsp dried rosemary or oregano

¼ cup cold-pressed extra virgin olive oil

*CARAMELISED ONION MIXTURE*

¼ cup cold-pressed extra virgin olive oil

4 large brown onions, thinly sliced

1 tbsp apple cider vinegar

2 tsp monk fruit sweetener or coconut sugar

Sea salt and freshly ground black pepper

*FILLING*

200 g (7 oz) feta

100 g (3½ oz) goat's cheese

¼ cup Greek yogurt

1 tbsp extra virgin olive oil

2 tbsp finely chopped fresh parsley, plus extra to serve

1 tbsp finely chopped fresh thyme leaves, plus extra to serve

1 tbsp finely chopped fresh chives

Sea salt and freshly ground black pepper

## METHOD

Preheat the oven to 180°C (350°F) and lightly grease a 22 cm (8.5-inch) tart dish.

To make the tart crust, combine the almond meal, bicarbonate of soda, sea salt and dried rosemary in a bowl. In a separate bowl, whisk the olive oil with 1 tablespoon cold water. Mix the wet and dry ingredients until a dough forms.

Press the dough evenly into the tart dish, covering the base and sides. (Ensure the tart crust is properly pressed.) Bake for 10 minutes to avoid sogginess, then remove from the oven to cool slightly.

To make the caramelised onions, heat the olive oil in a large frying pan over low heat. Add sliced onions and season with salt and pepper. Cook for about 30 minutes, stirring occasionally, until deeply caramelised.

Stir in the apple cider vinegar and monk fruit sweetener. Cook for another minute, then remove from heat.

To make the filling, in a medium bowl, mix the cheeses, Greek yogurt, olive oil, herbs, salt and pepper until smooth and creamy. Spread the herbed cheese mixture evenly over the pre-baked tart crust. Top with the caramelised onions.

Return to the oven and bake for an additional 15–20 minutes or until the crust is golden and the filling is set.

Garnish with extra fresh herbs. Serve warm or at room temperature with a crisp green salad on the side.

# CAULIFLOWER STEAKS WITH ZA'ATAR

These golden, spice-crusted cauliflower steaks are your inflammation-fighting champions on a plate. The vibrant za'atar blend is packed with anti-inflammatory compounds from oregano, thyme and sumac that help calm your body's inflammatory pathways, while the roasted cauliflower delivers sulforaphane, a powerful detoxing compound. Omega-3-rich walnuts and peppery rocket add extra anti-inflammatory punch, while the creamy goat's cheese provides easily digestible protein and probiotics.

**Serves 2**

## INGREDIENTS

1 large head of cauliflower, stems and leaves removed (or keep the leaves and roast with salt and olive oil)

2 garlic cloves, peeled and whole

3 tbsp extra virgin olive oil

3 tbsp ground paprika

1 tbsp sesame seeds

1 tbsp cumin seeds

1 tbsp lemon juice

4 tbsp za'atar

2 handfuls of rocket (arugula)

2 tbsp roughly chopped dried cranberries

2 tbsp roughly chopped walnuts

1 baby cucumber, skin peeled and sliced

20 g (¾ oz) goat's cheese

*DRESSING*

2 tbsp extra virgin olive oil

1 tbsp lemon juice

1 tsp Dijon mustard

Sea salt

## METHOD

Preheat the oven to 200°C (390°F). Line a baking tray with baking (parchment) paper.

Place the cauliflower upright on a chopping board, then slice off each end, about 1 cm (1/2 inch). Slice the cauliflower down the middle to create two flat steaks about 3–4 cm (1–1½ inches) thick.

Place the cauliflower and garlic on the lined tray, seasoning generously with olive oil and salt. Rub the paprika, sesame seeds, cumin seeds and lemon juice onto each steak then sprinkle with half the za'atar. Place tray in the oven and cook for 10 minutes.

Remove tray from oven and flip the steaks over. Sprinkle with the remaining za'atar and return to the oven. Bake for a further 10 minutes.

Meanwhile, prepare the salad and dressing. Toss the rocket, cranberries, walnuts and cucumber in a mixing bowl. Whisk together the dressing ingredients and pour over the salad. Divide the salad onto two serving plates.

When the cauliflower is ready, place onto the salad. Serve with crumbled goat's cheese and a final sprinkle of za'atar.

# SMOKED TROUT FRITTATA WITH PESTO & SALAD

A light yet satisfying frittata, packed with the smoky richness of trout, the freshness of zucchini (courgette) and the creamy tang of goat's cheese. The key to a perfect frittata is squeezing excess moisture from the zucchini to keep the texture light and airy. This frittata is just as delicious warm or cold, making it ideal for meal prep, and any leftover pesto keeps well in the fridge for up to a week.

**Serves 4**

## INGREDIENTS

6 large eggs

¼ cup almond milk (or milk of your choice)

1 medium zucchini (courgette), grated and squeezed of excess water

100 g (3½ oz) smoked trout, flaked

80 g (2¾ oz) soft goat's cheese, crumbled

2 tbsp finely chopped fresh chives

2 tbsp finely chopped fresh parsley

1 garlic clove, minced

½ tsp sea salt

¼ tsp freshly ground black pepper

1 tbsp extra virgin olive oil or butter (for cooking)

*PESTO*

1 cup fresh basil leaves

30 g (1 oz) toasted pine nuts (or walnuts)

1 small garlic clove

2 tbsp nutritional yeast

Juice of ½ lemon

Sea salt

⅓ cup extra virgin olive oil

*ROCKET & AVOCADO SALAD*

2 large handfuls of rocket

1 ripe avocado, sliced

½ small red onion, thinly sliced

30 g (1 oz) toasted pumpkin seeds (pepitas)

1 tbsp extra virgin olive oil

1 tbsp lemon juice

Sea salt and freshly ground black pepper

### METHOD

To make the pesto, blend the basil, toasted pine nuts, garlic, nutritional yeast, lemon juice and a pinch of salt in a food processor. Slowly drizzle in the olive oil, blending until smooth. Adjust seasoning as needed.

Preheat the oven to 180°C (350°F).

To make the frittata, whisk the eggs and almond milk in a large bowl. Season with salt and pepper. Stir in the grated zucchini, smoked trout, goat's cheese, herbs and garlic. Heat the olive oil in an ovenproof frying pan over medium heat. Pour the egg mixture into the pan and cook for 3–4 minutes until the edges start to set.

Transfer the pan to the oven and bake for 12–15 minutes or until the frittata is fully set and slightly golden.

To make the salad, toss the rocket, sliced avocado, red onion and toasted pumpkin seeds in a bowl. Drizzle with the olive oil and lemon juice, and season with salt and pepper.

When ready, slice the frittata and add a generous drizzle of homemade pesto. Serve alongside the rocket and avocado salad.

# LOW & SLOW BONE BROTH STEW

My deeply nourishing stew is loaded with medicinal bone broth, which supports gut lining repair, provides essential amino acids, and is a rich source of collagen to reduce inflammation and support joint health. Infused with warming spices, fresh herbs and citrus zest, it delivers healing benefits with a deep, comforting flavour. For best results, use high-quality grass-fed beef or free-range chicken. Adding apple cider vinegar helps extract more minerals from the bones, while searing the meat beforehand enhances richness. The stew tastes even better the next day, making it perfect for meal prep. Store leftovers in the fridge for up to 4 days or freeze for later.

**Serves 3**

## INGREDIENTS

- 300 g (10½ oz) grass-fed beef or free-range chicken, cubed
- 1 cup chopped carrots
- 1 cup chopped celery
- 1 small onion, finely chopped
- 2 cloves garlic, minced
- 1 tsp ground cumin
- 1 tsp ground turmeric
- ½ tsp ground cinnamon
- ½ tsp sea salt (or to taste)
- ¼ tsp freshly ground black pepper
- 2 cups bone broth (chicken or beef)
- 1 tbsp apple cider vinegar
- 1 bay leaf
- 1 sprig fresh rosemary
- 1 sprig fresh thyme
- ½ tsp lemon zest
- 1 tbsp chopped fresh parsley, to serve
- 1 tbsp extra virgin olive oil or ghee (for searing, optional)

## METHOD

If time allows, heat a tablespoon of olive oil in a pan over medium heat. Sear the beef or chicken for 2–3 minutes on each side until browned, then transfer to a slow cooker. This step enhances the depth of flavour.

Add the chopped carrots, celery and onion to the slow cooker, followed by the garlic, cumin, turmeric, cinnamon, salt and pepper.

Pour in the bone broth and apple cider vinegar, ensuring the ingredients are well covered. Add the bay leaf, rosemary and thyme. Cover and cook on low for 6–8 hours or high for 3–4 hours until the meat is tender and the flavours have developed fully.

Remove the bay leaf and herb stems. Stir in the lemon zest for a fresh, bright note. Taste and adjust seasoning if needed.

Ladle into bowls, garnish with fresh parsley and serve warm. This stew pairs well with cauliflower rice or quinoa for a more substantial meal.

# GLUTEN-FREE SALMON BURGERS

Serve these nourishing salmon burgers on slices of gluten-free oat and almond flour bread for a hearty, protein-rich meal. A creamy yogurt-herb sauce adds brightness, while fresh cucumber and lettuce bring a refreshing crunch.

***Cooking tip:*** *For extra texture, lightly toast the bread before assembling the burger.*

**Serves 2**

## INGREDIENTS

*SAUCE*

1 cup Greek yogurt

Drizzle of extra virgin olive oil

2 garlic cloves, minced

2 spring onions, chopped

1 tbsp capers (optional)

1 small chilli, chopped (optional)

Juice of 1 lemon plus 1 tsp lemon zest

Handful of fresh mint leaves

Handful of fresh dill

A few fresh basil leaves

Sea salt and freshly ground black pepper

*SALMON PATTIES*

200 g (7 oz) salmon fillets, chopped

1 heaped tbsp rice flour

Sea salt and freshly ground black pepper

1 tbsp sesame seeds (for texture)

*BREAD & TOPPINGS*

Extra virgin olive oil, for frying

4 slices Gluten-free oat and almond-flour bread (page 246)

½ cucumber, peeled and sliced

Iceberg lettuce, shredded

Fresh coriander (cilantro), to serve (optional)

Shaved aged goat's cheese (optional)

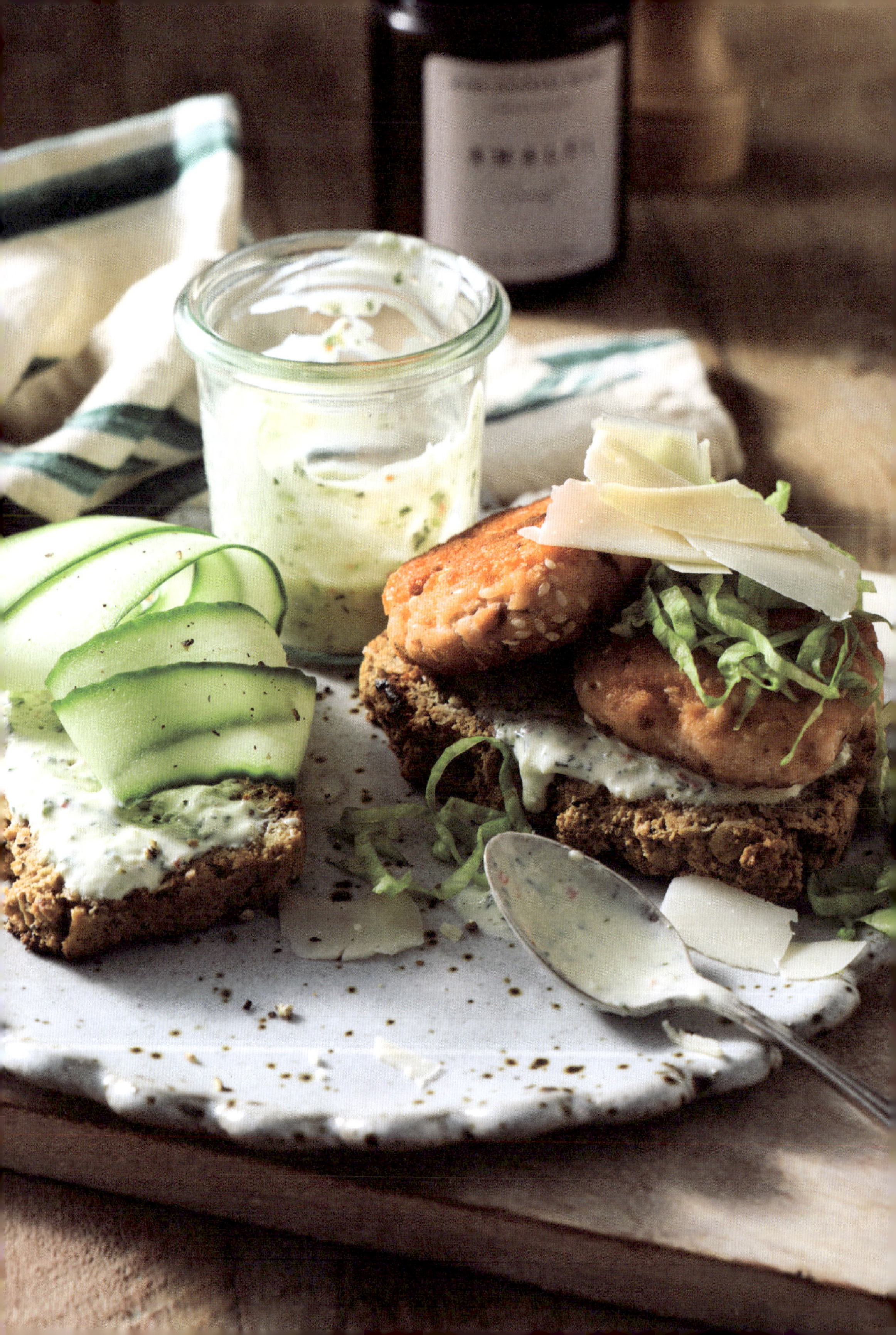

## METHOD

To prepare the yogurt sauce, combine all the ingredients in a blender or food processor. Blend until smooth and creamy. Set aside.

To make the salmon patties, add the chopped salmon, rice flour, and salt and pepper to taste to a food processor. Pulse until the mixture just comes together but still has some texture. Stir in the sesame seeds. Shape into four small patties.

Heat a drizzle of olive oil in a frying pan over medium heat. Cook the salmon patties for 3–4 minutes on each side until golden brown and cooked through. Remove from the pan.

To assemble the burgers, lightly toast the gluten-free bread slices. Spread a generous layer of the yogurt sauce on each slice. Top with shredded iceberg lettuce, cucumber slices and the salmon patties. Add shaved goat's cheese and fresh coriander (if using).

Serve the burgers open-faced or stack for a sandwich-style option. Pair with a simple side salad or roasted sweet potatoes for a complete meal.

### *STORAGE*

Store the yogurt sauce in the fridge for up to 3 days.

Refrigerate the salmon patties for up to 2 days.

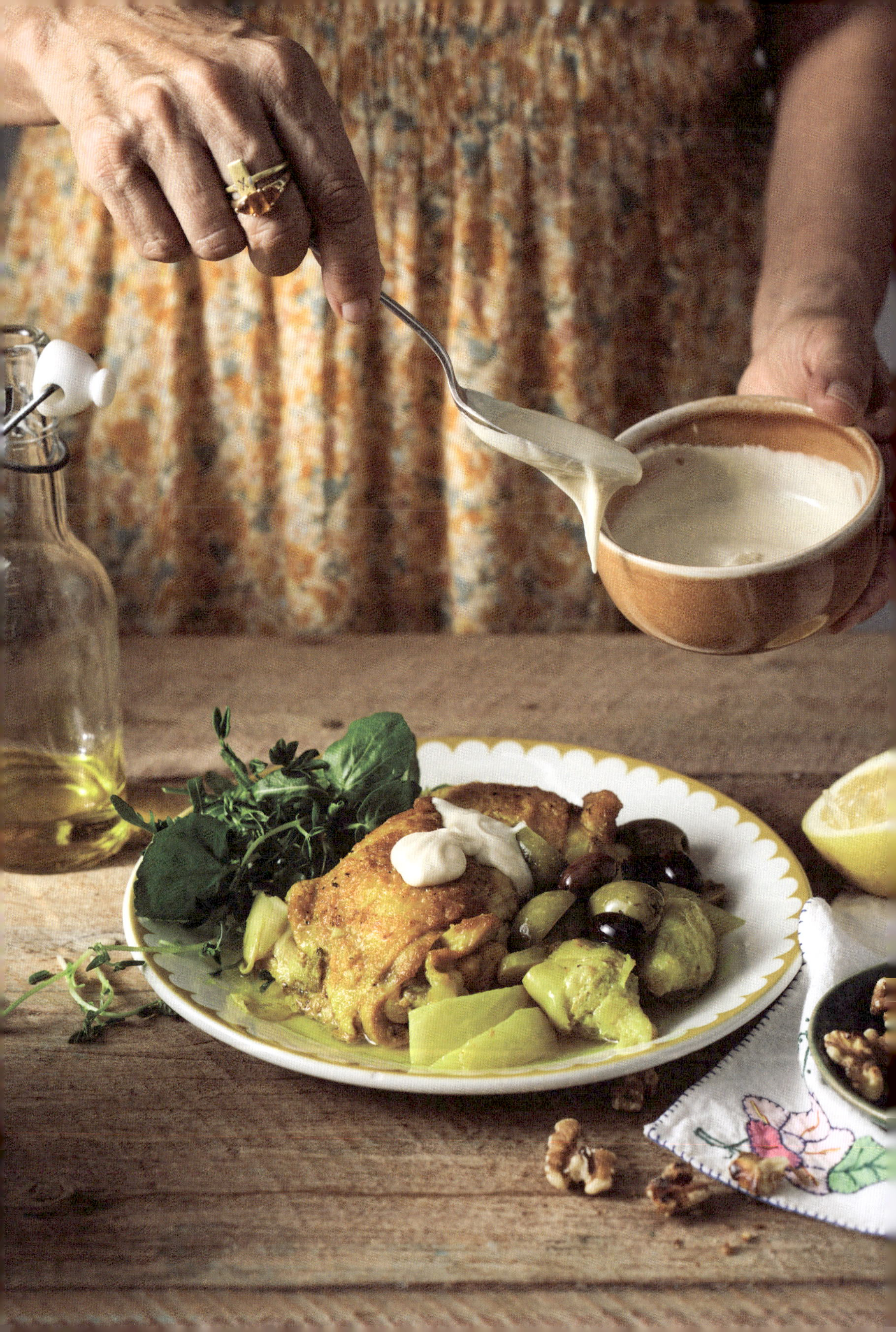

# LEMON-BRAISED CHICKEN WITH TAHINI DRIZZLE

This slow-cooked, Mediterranean-inspired one-pan meal champions the MAP principles. Bone-in chicken is gently braised with anti-inflammatory artichokes, fennel and citrus to maximise flavour without triggering harmful AGEs. A creamy lemon-tahini drizzle adds a boost of healthy fats, while a topping of fresh microgreens and chopped olives provide gut-friendly polyphenols. It's comfort food that's light, functional and deeply nourishing.

**Serves 3–4**

## INGREDIENTS

4 bone-in, skin-on organic chicken thighs

1 tsp ground turmeric

½ tsp ground cumin

¼ tsp freshly ground black pepper

Sea salt

1 tbsp extra virgin olive oil

1 small fennel bulb, sliced into wedges

1 cup artichoke hearts (frozen or jarred in brine, not oil), halved

3 cloves garlic, sliced

1 small lemon, thinly sliced

½ cup Slow-cooked chicken bone broth (page 247)

Juice of ½ lemon

*TAHINI DRIZZLE*

2 tbsp tahini

Juice of ½ lemon

1 tsp extra virgin olive oil

1 tbsp warm water (to loosen)

Sea salt

*TO SERVE*

½ cup microgreens (rocket/arugula, watercress or broccoli sprouts)

1 tbsp finely chopped black or green olives

Sprinkle of toasted crushed walnuts or hemp seeds (optional)

### METHOD

Pat the chicken dry and season with the turmeric, cumin, pepper and a pinch of salt. In a heavy pan or Dutch oven, heat the olive oil over medium–low heat. Add the chicken skin-side down and let it gently brown for 8–10 minutes without flipping – just enough to render some fat without high heat. Flip and sear the other side for 2–3 minutes.

Add the fennel, artichoke hearts, garlic and lemon slices to the pan, tucking them around the chicken. Pour in the broth and lemon juice. Bring to a gentle simmer, cover, and reduce heat to low. Let it cook slowly for 40–50 minutes until the chicken is tender and cooked through.

While it cooks, make the tahini drizzle. Whisk together the tahini, lemon juice, olive oil, warm water and a pinch of salt in a small bowl.

When the chicken is ready, let it rest for a few minutes off the heat. Spoon over the tahini drizzle, then top with the microgreens, chopped olives and walnuts (if using) just before serving.

# SOBA NOODLES WITH ZUCCHINI & MANGO

**Serves 2**

## INGREDIENTS

225 g (8 oz) soba noodles

1 tbsp extra virgin olive oil

2 cloves garlic, minced

2 medium zucchini (courgettes), sliced into thin strips

1 fresh red chilli, seeded and finely chopped

1 tsp dried oregano

1 tsp dried rosemary

½ tsp freshly ground black pepper

Sea salt

1 large ripe mango, diced

2 tbsp lemon juice

Zest of 1 large lemon

½ medium red onion, thinly sliced

1 tbsp tahini (optional)

Chopped fresh parsley or coriander, to garnish

Toasted sesame seeds, to garnish (optional)

## METHOD

Bring a large pot of salted water to a boil. Cook the soba noodles according to the package instructions (about 4–5 minutes). Drain and rinse under cold water to remove excess starch.

Meanwhile, in a large frying pan, heat the olive oil over medium heat. Add the garlic and sauté for 1 minute until fragrant. Add the sliced zucchini and cook until they start to soften, about 4 minutes. Add the chopped fresh chilli and cook for another minute, stirring occasionally. Season with the oregano, rosemary, pepper and a pinch of salt.

In a large mixing bowl, mix the diced mango with a squeeze of lemon juice to prevent browning. Combine the cooked soba noodles, sautéed zucchini and red onion. If using tahini, whisk it with a little water to thin it out, then drizzle over the noodles.

Serve the noodles garnished with fresh herbs and toasted sesame seeds (if using). Serve piled onto a plate.

# ZUCCHINI LINGUINE WITH CREAMY GREEN PESTO

A refreshing, anti-inflammatory take on pasta night – this dish replaces traditional pasta with light zucchini (courgette) linguine and swaps heavy sauces for a protein-rich, creamy pesto made with cottage cheese and walnuts. Roasted shredded kale adds crunch, fibre and earthy depth, while parmesan brings richness and balance. This MAP-friendly dinner is easy on the gut, low in AGEs and packed with phytonutrients for cellular health.

**Serves 2**

## INGREDIENTS

1 heaped cup kale leaves, finely shredded (stems removed)

3 tsp extra virgin olive oil

Sea salt

2 large zucchini (courgettes), spiralised or julienned into linguine

Extra grated parmesan, to serve

Lemon zest or microgreens, to serve (optional)

*CREAMY PESTO*

½ cup full-fat cottage cheese

¼ cup chopped walnuts

¼ cup grated parmesan

1 small garlic clove

Juice of ½ lemon

2 tbsp extra virgin olive oil

Small handful of fresh basil or parsley

Sea salt and freshly ground black pepper

## METHOD

Toss the shredded kale with 2 teaspoons olive oil and salt. Spread onto a lined baking tray and roast at 160°C (320°F) for 10–12 minutes, stirring once, until crisp but not browned.

To make the creamy pesto, blend all the ingredients in a blender or food processor. Add a splash of warm water as needed for consistency.

Warm the remaining olive oil in a large pan over low heat. Add the zucchini noodles with a pinch of salt and gently cook for 2–3 minutes, just until tender.

Remove from the heat and toss the noodles with the pesto until well coated. Serve topped with the roasted kale, extra parmesan, and lemon zest or microgreens (if using).

# ALMOND-MEAL PIZZA WITH GOAT'S CHEESE & CARAMELISED ONIONS

This MAP-friendly pizza delivers all the comfort of a classic without the inflammation. The almond-meal base is fibre-rich, blood glucose-friendly and full of healthy fats. Goat's cheese adds a creamy contrast to the sweet caramelised onions, while fresh rocket brings peppery brightness and digestive support. Baked at a moderate temperature to minimise AGE formation, this is a gut-friendly, hormone-supportive dinner that feels indulgent yet deeply nourishing.

**Serves 2**

## INGREDIENTS

*ALMOND BASE*

1¼ cups almond meal

1 tbsp ground linseeds (flaxseeds)

½ tsp baking powder

Sea salt

1 egg

2 tbsp extra virgin olive oil

1 tbsp filtered water

¾ cup goat's cheese

1 large handful rocket (arugula)

Fresh thyme or oregano leaves (optional)

Freshly ground black pepper

*CARAMELISED ONIONS*

2 small red onions, thinly sliced

1 tsp extra virgin olive oil

Sea salt

1 tsp balsamic vinegar

## METHOD

Preheat the oven to 180°C (350°F).

To make the almond base, mix the almond meal, linseeds, baking powder and a pinch of salt in a bowl. Add the egg, olive oil and water then stir into a sticky dough. Roll out dough between two pieces of baking (parchment) paper into a thin round (about 0.5 cm/¼ inch). Place on a baking tray and peel off the top layer.

Bake the base for 12–15 minutes until golden and firm. Remove from oven and let cool slightly.

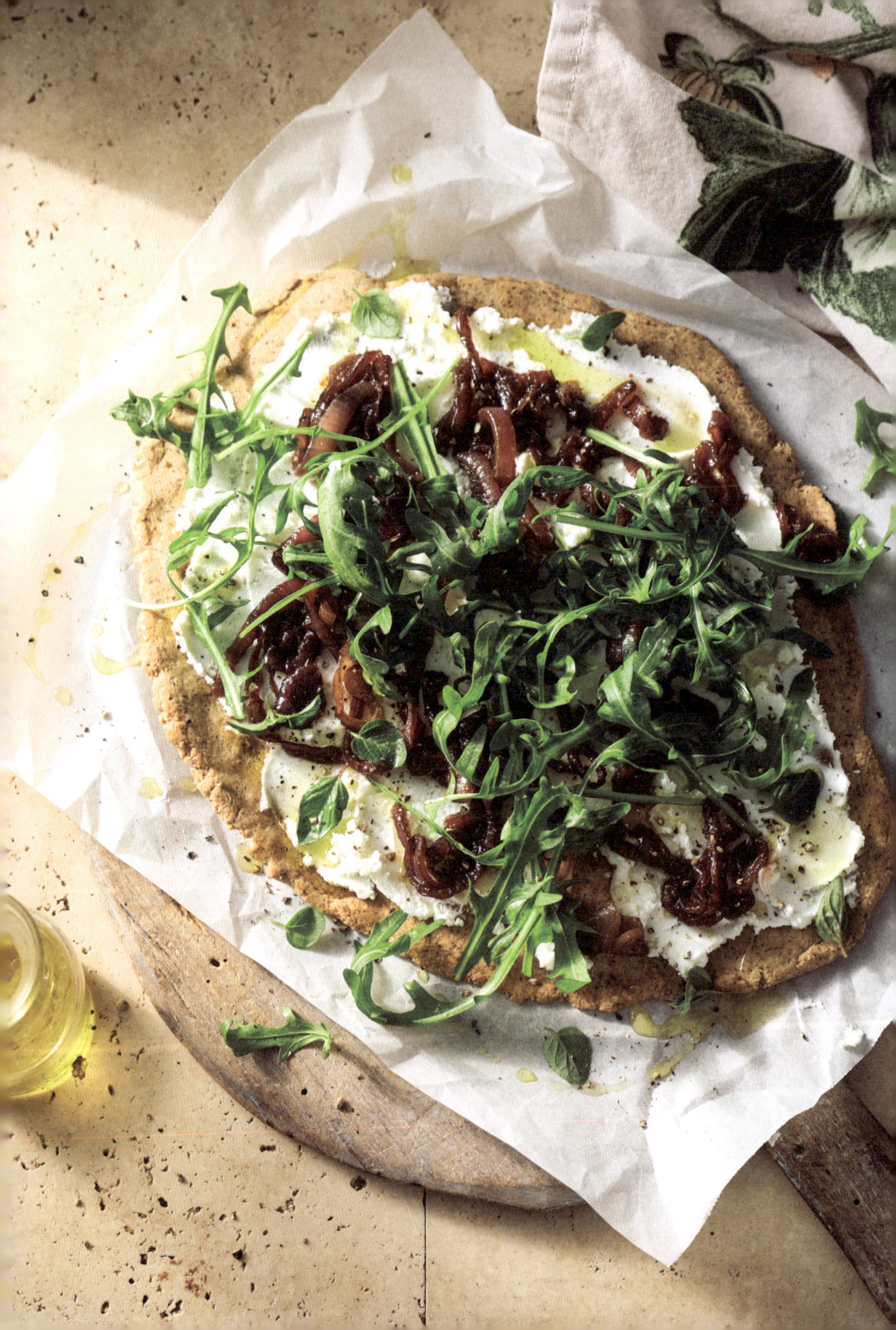

Meanwhile, heat a pan over low heat. Add the onions, olive oil and a pinch of salt. Cook slowly for 15–20 minutes, stirring occasionally. Add balsamic vinegar and cook for 2–3 more minutes until soft and caramelised.

Spread the goat's cheese over the cooled base. Season with salt and pepper. Top with the warm caramelised onions. Return pizza to the oven for 5–7 minutes to just warm through if desired.

Top with the fresh rocket and herbs. Drizzle with some olive oil and a grind of black pepper to serve.

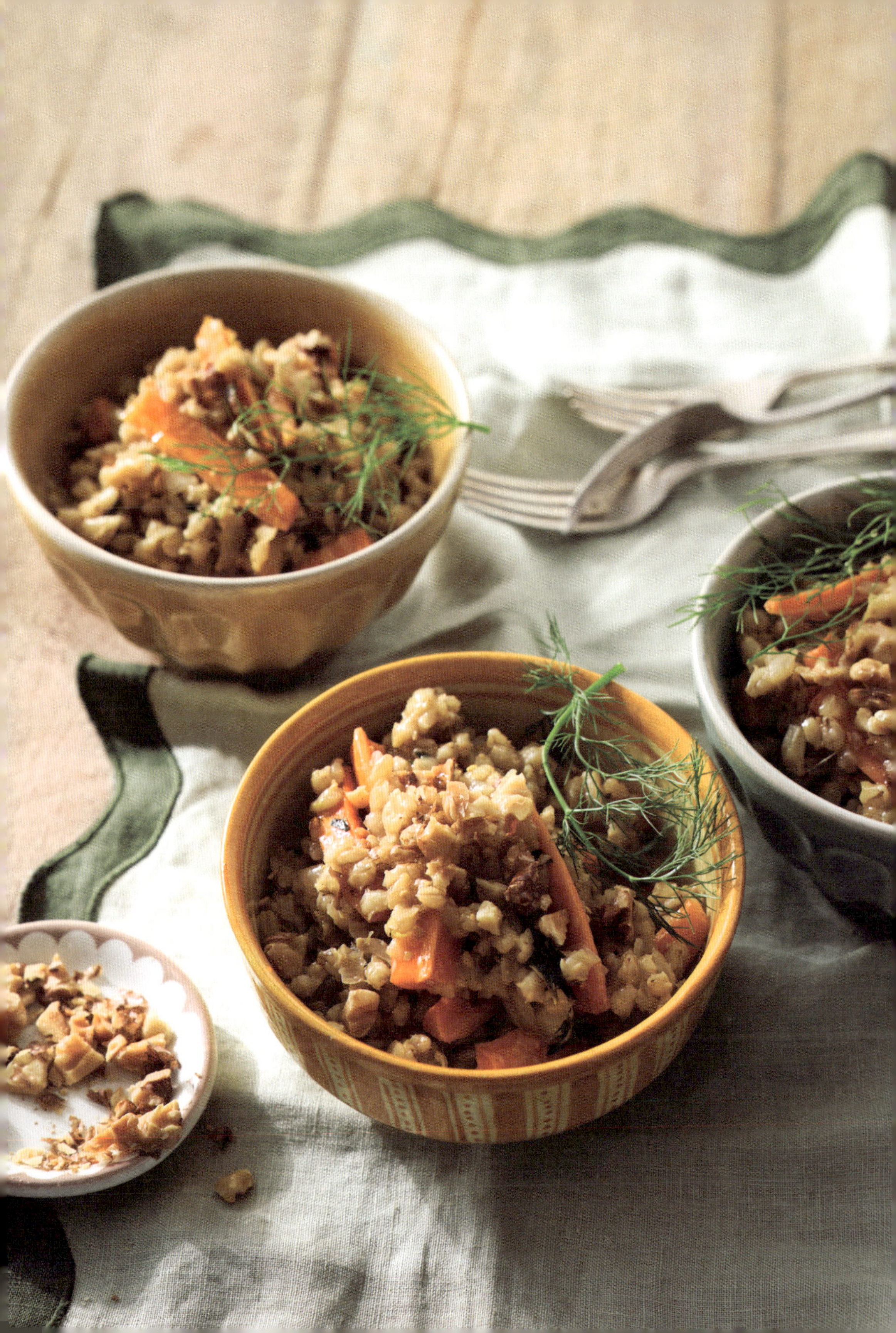

# BARLEY & ROASTED CARROT RISOTTO

Barley provides beta-glucan fibre for gut health and blood glucose balance, while roasted carrots offer carotenoids and sweetness. Toasted walnuts add crunch and omega-3s. Cooked low and slow to preserve nutrients and minimise AGEs.

**Serves 2–3**

## INGREDIENTS

4 medium carrots, peeled and cut into batons

2 tbsp extra virgin olive oil, plus extra to serve

1 tsp fresh thyme leaves

Sea salt and freshly ground black pepper

1 small leek, white part only, finely chopped

1 small fennel bulb, finely chopped (reserve fronds for garnish)

¾ cup hulled barley, soaked for 6–8 hours (or overnight), then rinsed and drained

1 garlic clove, minced

750 ml (26 fl oz) low-sodium vegetable stock (broth)

Juice and zest of ½ lemon

Small handful of fresh mint leaves, chopped

¼ cup walnuts, lightly toasted and roughly chopped

## METHOD

Preheat the oven to 170°C (340°F).

Toss the carrots with 1 tablespoon olive oil, salt to taste and thyme. Spread on a baking tray and roast for 25–30 minutes until golden and tender.

Meanwhile, in a large pot, heat the remaining olive oil over low heat. Add the leek and fennel, cooking gently for 10 minutes until softened. Add the barley and garlic, stirring to coat.

Pour in half the stock. Cover the pot and simmer gently, stirring occasionally. Gradually add more stock as it absorbs – this will take about 40–55 minutes until the barley is plump and tender with a slight chew.

Stir in the roasted carrots and lemon zest. Season with salt and pepper. Remove from heat and fold in the mint and lemon juice.

Serve warm, topped with the toasted walnuts, reserved fennel fronds and a drizzle of olive oil.

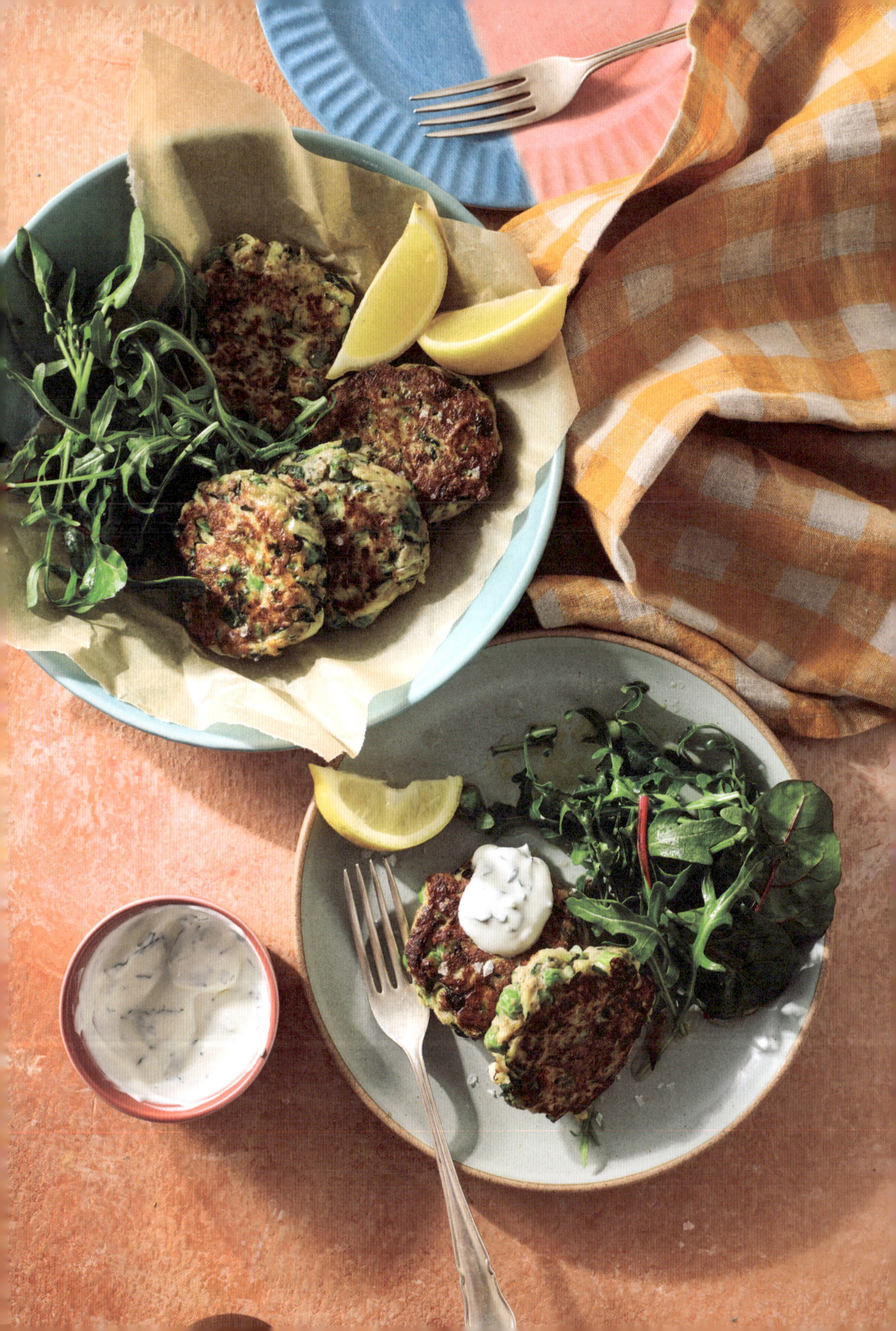

# SARDINE, ZUCCHINI & PEA FRITTERS WITH MINT YOGURT

These savoury fritters are rich in omega-3s, fibre, and plant compounds that support brain, gut, and hormone health. Sardines are a MAP superfood – low in mercury, high in calcium and anti-inflammatory fats – while zucchini (courgette) and peas add gentle fibre and prebiotics. Pan-fried over low–medium heat and served with a cooling mint yogurt and a crisp side of lemon-dressed leaves, this is a balanced lunch or light dinner that's as satisfying as it is nourishing.

**Serves 2**

## INGREDIENTS

1 small zucchini (courgette), grated and squeezed of excess water

½ cup peas (fresh or thawed from frozen)

1 small tin sardines in olive oil (about 90 g/3 oz), drained and flaked

2 tbsp buckwheat flour or almond meal

2 tbsp finely chopped spring onions (scallions) or chives

1 tbsp chopped fresh parsley

1 egg

½ tsp ground cumin

Sea salt and freshly ground black pepper

Extra virgin olive oil spray (optional, for air frying)

*MINT YOGURT*

⅓ cup full-fat Greek yogurt

1 tbsp finely chopped fresh mint

Juice of ¼ lemon

Pinch of sea salt

*LEMON-DRESSED GREENS*

2 handfuls mixed leafy greens (rocket/arugula, baby spinach, watercress)

Juice of ½ lemon

1 tsp extra virgin olive oil

Sea salt

## METHOD

Combine the zucchini, peas, sardines, flour, spring onions, parsley, egg and cumin in a bowl. Season with salt and pepper, mix well, and let sit for 5–10 minutes to firm up slightly.

Form the mixture into six small patties and place on a tray or plate lined with baking (parchment) paper.

Preheat the air fryer to 180°C (350°F).

Lightly spray or brush the fritters with olive oil (if using). Air-fry for 10–12 minutes, flipping halfway, until golden and cooked through. Alternatively, to pan-fry, heat 1–2 tablespoons olive oil in a non-stick frying pan (skillet) over medium–low heat. Cook the fritters for 4–5 minutes on each side until golden brown and cooked through.

In the meantime, make the mint yogurt. Stir together all the ingredients and chill.

To make the lemon-dressed greens, toss the salad leaves with the lemon juice, olive oil and a pinch of sea salt just before serving.

Serve the warm fritters with the mint yogurt and lemony leaves on the side.

# SLOW-COOKED LAMB SHOULDER WITH BUTTER BEANS & CAVOLO NERO

Crafted to fit the MAP diet, this dish supports gut health, balances inflammation and delivers sustained nourishment through whole, minimally processed ingredients and gentle cooking methods. The lamb provides complete amino acids and B vitamins essential for neurotransmitter production. The iron-rich cavolo nero supports healthy oxygen delivery to your brain, and the butter beans offer magnesium and folate that help maintain calm neural pathways and cognitive function. The bright orange-herb dressing adds anti-inflammatory vitamin C and polyphenols.

**Serves 4–6**

## INGREDIENTS

1.2–1.5 kg lamb shoulder, bone-in

Sea salt and freshly ground black pepper

1 tbsp extra virgin olive oil

1 onion, sliced

4 garlic cloves, smashed

1 tbsp chopped fresh rosemary (or 1 tsp dried)

Zest of 1 orange

Juice of 1 lemon

1 cup filtered water or low-sodium vegetable stock (broth)

### *ORANGE-HERB DRESSING*

Zest and juice of ½ orange

2 tbsp extra virgin olive oil

1 tbsp finely chopped fresh parsley

1 tsp finely chopped fresh oregano or thyme

½ tsp Dijon mustard (optional, for emulsification)

Pinch of sea salt

### *CAVOLO NERO & BEANS*

1 bunch cavolo nero (Tuscan kale), stems removed and leaves roughly chopped

1 tbsp extra virgin olive oil

Juice of ½ lemon

Pinch of sea salt

1 can butter beans, drained and rinsed

### METHOD

Preheat the oven to 150°C (300°F). Pat the lamb dry and season well with salt and pepper.

In a large ovenproof pot or Dutch oven, heat the olive oil over medium heat. Sear the lamb on all sides until lightly golden. Remove and set aside.

In the same pot, sauté the onion and garlic until soft. Stir in the rosemary and orange zest, then return lamb to the pot. Pour in the lemon juice and water, scraping up any browned bits from the bottom of the pot.

Cover tightly and roast in the oven for 3½–4 hours, basting once or twice, until the lamb is tender and pulls apart with a fork.

To make the orange-herb dressing, whisk together all the ingredients. Set aside.

About 20 minutes before serving, make the cavolo nero and beans. Steam or sauté the cavolo nero with olive oil, lemon juice and salt until just tender. Stir through the butter beans to warm.

Serve the shredded lamb on a bed of cavolo nero and beans, drizzled generously with the dressing.

# DESSERTS, SNACKS AND SAVOURIES

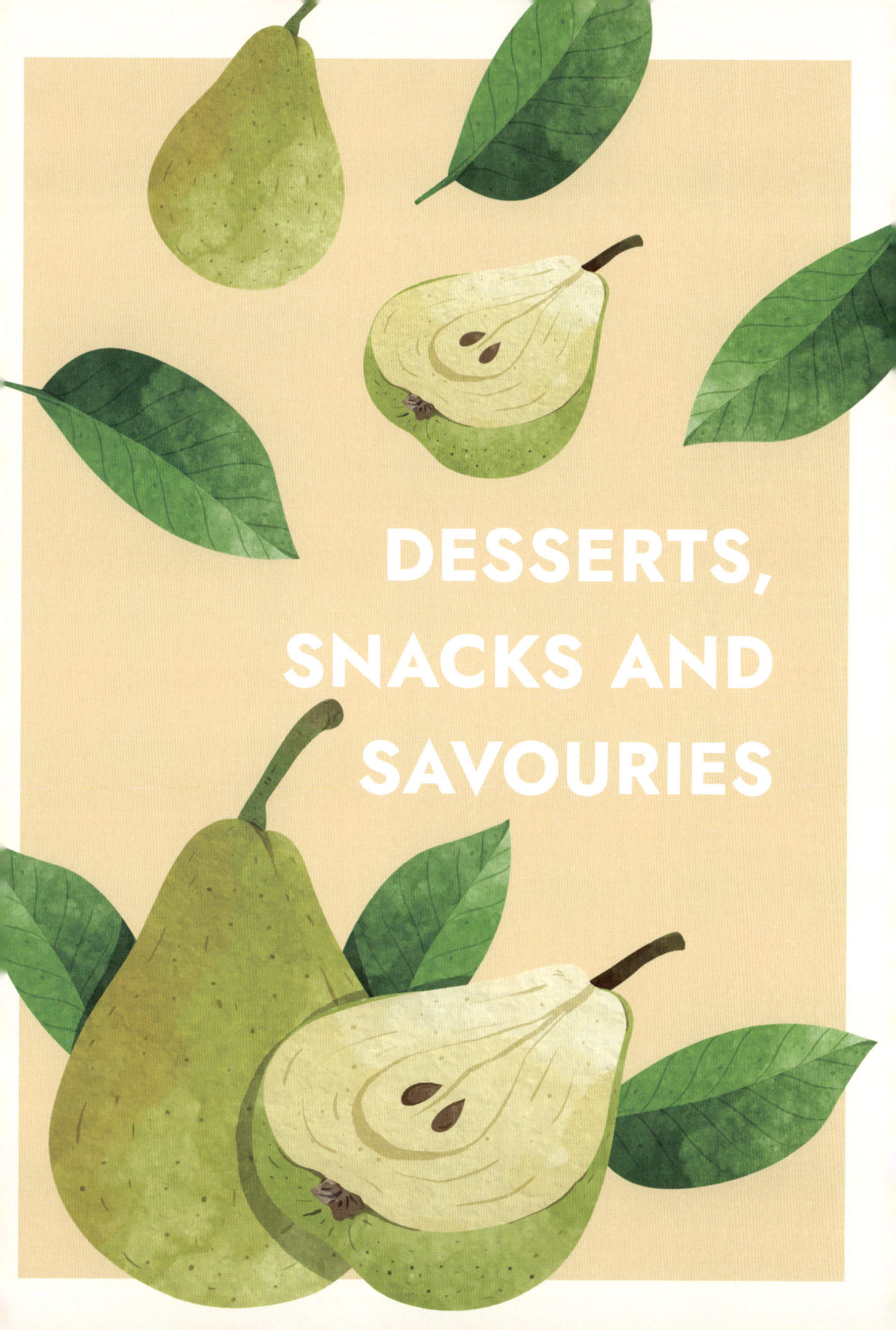

# INFLAMMATION-FIGHTING TRAIL MIX

A simple yet nutrient-packed snack that's filled with anti-inflammatory nuts and seeds, this trail mix is rich in omega-3 fatty acids and antioxidants. It supports gut health, brain function and energy levels throughout the day.

***Cooking tip:*** *Lightly toast in a dry pan over medium heat for 2–3 minutes.*

**Makes 1½ cups**

## INGREDIENTS

½ cup walnuts
½ cup almonds
2 tbsp pumpkin seeds (pepitas)
2 tbsp linseeds (flaxseeds)
2 tbsp dried blueberries
2 tbsp cacao nibs

## METHOD

Mix all the ingredients in a bowl. Store in an airtight container and enjoy as a snack.

# GOLDEN ENERGY BALLS

These energy balls combine the anti-inflammatory power of turmeric with healthy fats, fibre, and gut-friendly prebiotics and probiotics. The coconut and almonds provide sustained energy, while turmeric helps reduce oxidative stress and inflammation. Adding the Love Your Gut Synbiotic Powder enhances digestion and supports a balanced gut microbiome.

***Cooking tip:*** *Chilling the mixture before rolling makes shaping easier.*

**Makes 30 small balls (or 15 large)**

### INGREDIENTS

1 cup linseed (flaxseed) or almond meal

½ cup shredded coconut, plus extra for rolling

¼ cup yacon or maple syrup

2 tbsp chopped nuts (walnuts or pistachios)

1 tbsp Love Your Gut Synbiotic Powder

1 tbsp tahini or almond butter

2 medjool dates, pitted and blended

2 tsp ground turmeric

1 tsp coconut oil

1 tsp grated fresh ginger

1 tsp vanilla extract

½ tsp ground cinnamon

¼ tsp sea salt

### METHOD

Blend all the ingredients in a food processor until a sticky dough forms. Add a teaspoon of water as needed to help it come together. Chill the mixture in the fridge for 10–15 minutes to firm up.

Roll mixture into small balls and coat with extra shredded coconut. Refrigerate for at least 30 minutes before serving. Store in an airtight container in the fridge for up to a week.

# SARDINE CRACKERS

My protein-packed crackers are like portable brain fuel that let you crunch your way to mental clarity. The omega-3-rich sardines and linseeds (flaxseed) double down on your brain's favourite fatty acids, plus linseeds provide lignans that support hormonal balance. Almonds adds magnesium and vitamin E to protect your brain cells from oxidative stress, and fresh parsley is loaded with folate and vitamin K for healthy neurotransmitter production. Pair it with my Healthy tzatziki dip (opposite page) to support your gut–brain axis, making a satisfying snack that helps your nervous system find its natural rhythm while giving you sustained energy.

***Cooking tip:*** *Use a fork to press the cracker dough thinly for crispier crackers.*

**Serves 2**

## INGREDIENTS

2 cans (220 g/7¾ oz in total) sardines in olive oil, mashed

½ cup almond flour

½ cup linseed (flaxseed) meal

1 tbsp lemon juice

1 tbsp chopped fresh parsley

## METHOD

Mix all the ingredients into a dough. Roll out, cut into cracker shapes and bake at 180°C (350°F) for 15 minutes.

# HEALTHY TZATZIKI DIP

***Cooking tip:*** *For an extra twist, you can add a tablespoon of tahini or a small drizzle of maple syrup for a subtle sweetness.*

**Makes 1½ cups**

## INGREDIENTS

1 medium cucumber

1 cup Greek yogurt

1–2 cloves garlic, minced (adjust to taste)

1 tbsp extra virgin olive oil

1 tbsp fresh lemon juice

1–2 tsp chopped fresh dill (or 1 tsp dried)

½ tsp sea salt (or to taste)

¼ tsp freshly ground black pepper (or to taste)

Pinch of ground cumin or smoked paprika (optional)

## METHOD

Grate the cucumber and squeeze out any excess moisture using a clean cloth or paper towel (kitchen paper). This will help keep the dip thick.

In a bowl, combine the Greek yogurt, grated cucumber, garlic, olive oil, lemon juice, dill, salt and pepper. Stir until smooth and well combined.

Let the dip sit in the fridge for at least 30 minutes. This helps the flavours meld and makes the dip extra refreshing. Serve with ground cumin (if using).

# COCONUT YOGURT BOWL WITH FIGS & PASSIONFRUIT

The combination of creamy yogurt and almond butter, topped with fresh figs and passionfruit, creates a deliciously satisfying and gut-friendly breakfast or snack. A sprinkle of hemp seeds adds extra protein and omega-3s, while a touch of sea salt enhances the flavours.

**Serves 1**

## INGREDIENTS

1 cup coconut yogurt (unsweetened)

1 scoop Supercharged Food Vanilla Protein Powder (or protein powder of your choice)

1 tbsp almond butter

2 fresh figs, sliced

1 passionfruit, pulp scooped out

1 tsp hemp seeds

Sea salt

## METHOD

In a bowl, mix the coconut yogurt with the protein powder until smooth and well combined.

Swirl in the almond butter. Top with sliced figs and passionfruit pulp. Sprinkle with hemp seeds and a pinch of sea salt. Serve immediately and enjoy.

---

### *OPTIONAL ADDITIONS*

Add a handful of granola or toasted coconut flakes for extra crunch.

Stir in some chia seeds for additional fibre and omega-3s.

# MEDJOOL DATES STUFFED WITH GOAT'S CHEESE & WALNUTS

A naturally sweet, fibre-rich treat that's balanced with creamy goat's cheese and crunchy walnuts. These stuffed dates offer gut-friendly benefits and are packed with anti-inflammatory fats and polyphenols.

**Serves 2 (makes 6 stuffed dates)**

## INGREDIENTS

6 medjool dates

3 tbsp soft goat's cheese

6 walnut halves

Pinch of cinnamon or sumac (optional)

## METHOD

Make a small slit in each date and gently open. Remove the seed. Fill each with half a tablespoon of goat's cheese and top with a walnut half. Sprinkle with cinnamon or sumac (if using). Chill before serving.

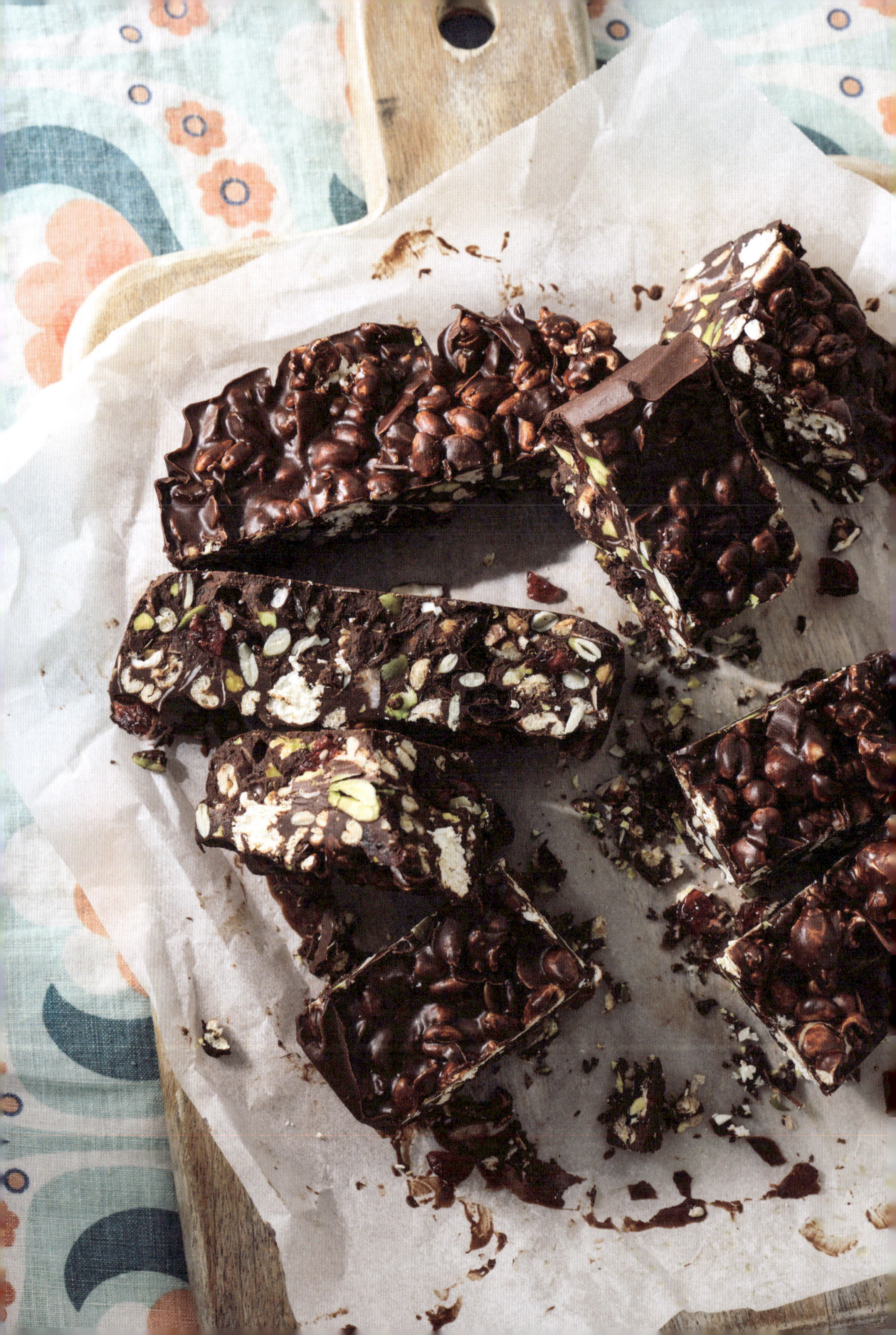

# RASPBERRY-PISTACHIO ROCKY-ROAD BARS

**Makes 10 bars**

## INGREDIENTS

200 g (7 oz) dark chocolate (85% cacao or higher), melted

¼ cup coconut oil, melted

2 tbsp almond butter (or tahini for extra creaminess)

1 tbsp pure maple syrup (optional)

½ tsp vanilla extract

1 cup popcorn or puffed cereal of your choice

½ cup pistachios, roughly chopped

½ cup dried raspberries

¼ cup coconut flakes (unsweetened)

¼ cup pumpkin seeds (pepitas)

2 tbsp cacao nibs

½ tsp sea salt

## METHOD

Line a small baking dish with baking (parchment) paper.

Melt the chocolate and coconut oil in a heatproof bowl over a double boiler or in short bursts in the microwave. Stir until smooth.

Stir in the almond butter, maple syrup (if using) and vanilla until well combined. Fold in the popcorn, pistachios, raspberries, coconut flakes, pumpkin seeds, cacao nibs and sea salt. Mix gently to coat everything in the chocolate mixture.

Pour the mixture into the prepared dish and spread evenly. Chill in the fridge for at least 1 hour (or 30 minutes in the freezer) until firm.

Slice into bars. Store in the fridge for up to 2 weeks, or freezer for 2–3 months.

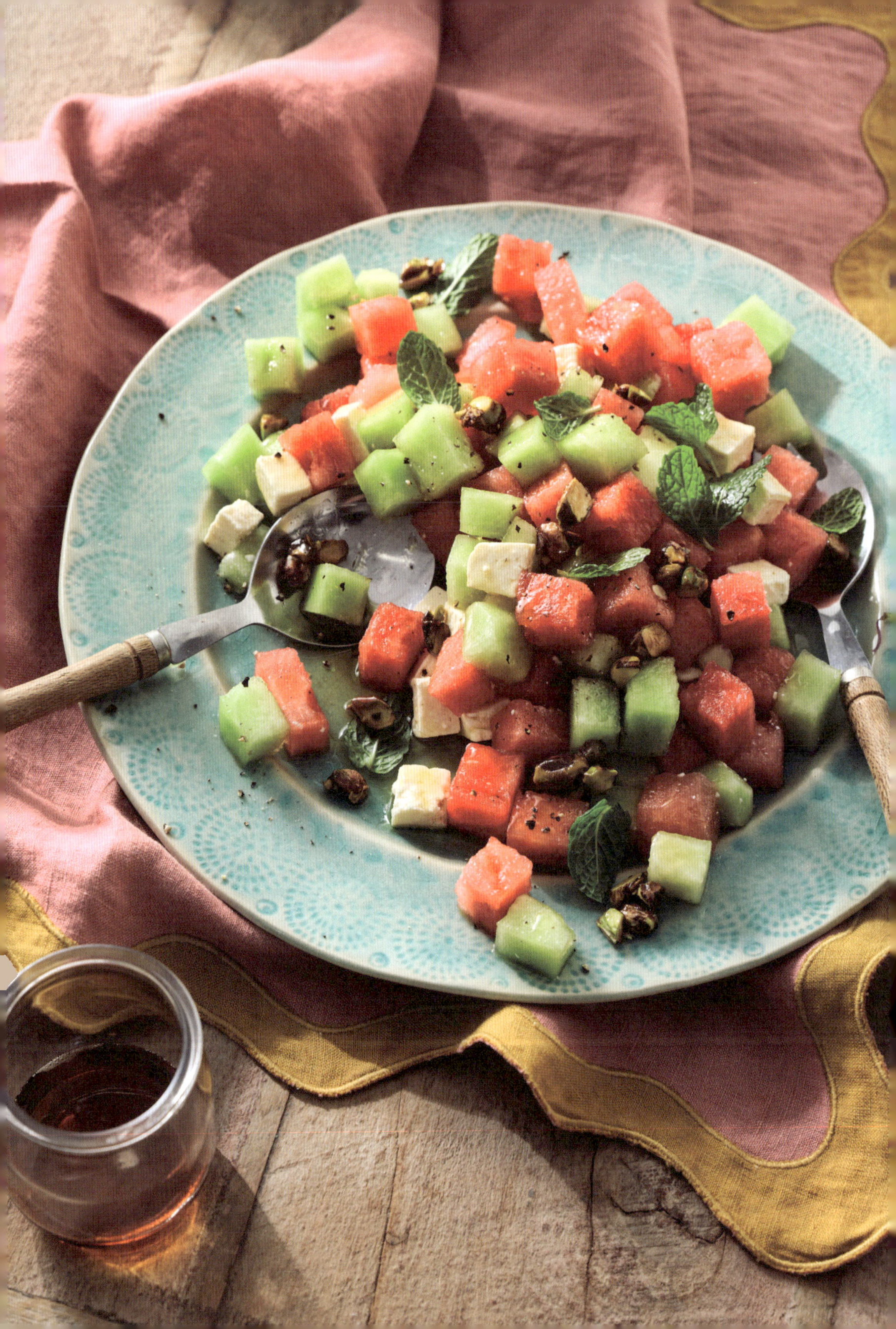

# FETA & MELON MOSAIC WITH MAPLE PISTACHIOS

This refreshing, antioxidant-rich snack or starter pairs the hydrating sweetness of melon with the probiotic richness of feta and the crunch of maple-glazed pistachios. Rich in vitamin C, beneficial fats and polyphenols, this dish brings together key MAP principles in one colourful, flavour-packed plate.

**Serves 4**

## INGREDIENTS

1 cup watermelon, diced into small cubes
1 cup honeydew melon, diced
80 g (2¾ oz) feta, cut into small cubes
2 tbsp raw pistachios, roughly chopped
1½ tsp maple syrup
1 tsp extra virgin olive oil (optional)
A few fresh mint leaves, torn, to serve
Freshly ground black pepper, to serve

## METHOD

Lightly toast the chopped pistachios in a dry frying pan (skillet) over low heat for 2–3 minutes, stirring regularly. Once fragrant, drizzle over 1 teaspoon maple syrup and stir for another 30–60 seconds until the pistachios are glossy and just beginning to caramelise. Transfer to baking (parchment) paper to cool.

Arrange the melon and feta cubes on a serving plate in a mosaic or scatter pattern.

Once the pistachios have cooled slightly and hardened, sprinkle them over the melon and feta. Drizzle with the remaining maple syrup and a touch of extra virgin olive oil (if using). Top with fresh mint leaves and some black pepper just before serving.

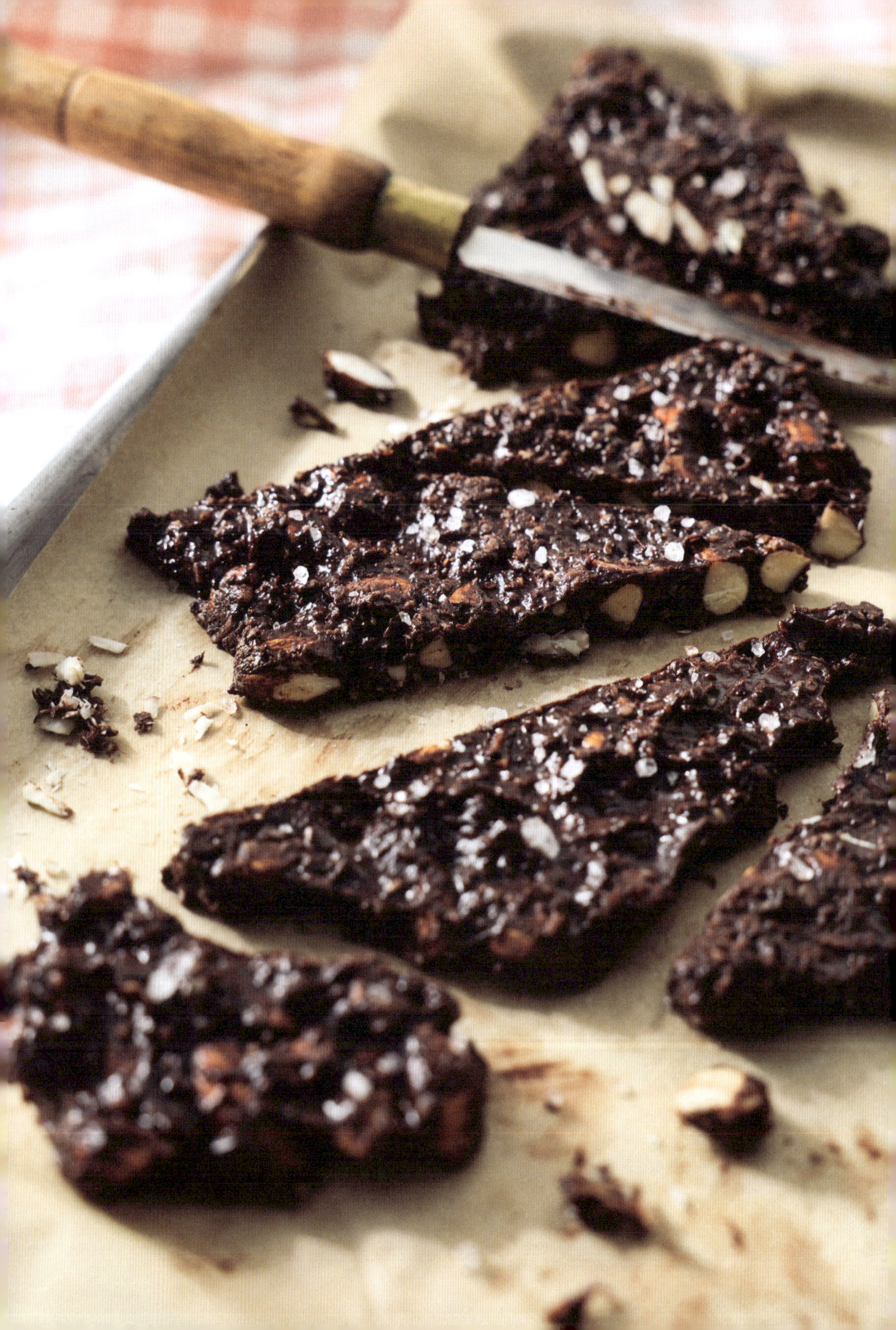

# ALMOND-CACAO CRUNCH BARK WITH HEMP SEEDS

This satisfying, no-bake snack is loaded with healthy fats, magnesium-rich cacao and omega-3s from hemp seeds. It's rich in antioxidants and provides a gentle energy lift – perfect for an afternoon pick-me-up or a nourishing sweet treat. This bark aligns beautifully with the MAP approach by balancing texture, taste and nutrient density.

**Makes 1 tray (about 12 pieces)**

## INGREDIENTS

2 tbsp almond butter
2 tbsp extra virgin coconut oil
2 tbsp maple or yacon syrup
3 tbsp raw cacao powder
Sea salt
1 cup raw almonds, roughly chopped
¼ cup hemp seeds
¼ cup shredded coconut (optional)
2 tbsp cacao nibs
Flaky sea salt, to garnish

## METHOD

Line a small baking tray with baking (parchment) paper.

In a small saucepan over low heat, melt the almond butter, coconut oil and maple syrup together. Stir in the cacao powder and a pinch of salt until smooth.

In a bowl, mix the almonds, hemp seeds, shredded coconut (if using) and cacao nibs. Pour the chocolate mixture over the dry ingredients and mix until evenly coated. Spread the mixture onto the lined tray, pressing it down evenly to form a thin bark layer. Sprinkle with a little flaky sea salt. Freeze for 1 hour or until solid.

Once set, break into shards and store in an airtight container in the fridge or freezer.

# BAKED ARTICHOKE & SPINACH DIP WITH BITTER LEAVES

Packed with fibre, healthy fats and polyphenols, this creamy, warming dip is slow-baked to protect delicate nutrients and support your digestion.

**Serves 4 (as a snack or starter)**

### INGREDIENTS

1½ cups cooked artichoke hearts (jarred in brine or frozen and thawed), chopped

2 cups baby spinach, chopped

1 cup Greek yogurt (sheep's or goat's for enhanced digestibility)

¼ cup soft goat's cheese or crumbled feta

1 tbsp extra virgin olive oil

1 small garlic clove, grated or finely minced

Zest of ½ lemon

1 tbsp lemon juice

2 tsp nutritional yeast (optional)

Sea salt and freshly ground black pepper

Handful of endive and radicchio leaves, to serve

Spiced nut & seed dukkah sprinkle, to serve (optional, page 248)

### METHOD

Preheat the oven to 150°C (300°F).

In a mixing bowl, combine the chopped artichoke hearts, spinach, yogurt, goat's cheese, olive oil, garlic, and lemon zest and juice. Season with salt and pepper, and stir until well mixed.

Transfer to a small baking dish and smooth the top. Cover with foil and bake low and slow for about 30–40 minutes, until warmed through and slightly golden on the edges. Remove foil for the final 10 minutes if you want a lightly caramelised top.

While the dip is baking, prepare your serving platter. Arrange endive and radicchio leaves around the edge of the dish in alternating layers, forming a floral-like ring.

Once the dip is ready, serve it warm in the centre of the bitter leaf ring. Drizzle with olive oil and top with dukkah (if using).

# RESVERATROL-RICH BERRY COMPOTE

This antioxidant-packed berry compote is rich in resveratrol, a powerful polyphenol with anti-inflammatory and longevity-promoting benefits. Blueberries, blackberries and grapes provide a natural sweetness, while warming spices and citrus zest enhance flavour and digestion. Perfect as a topping for yogurt, porridge or pancakes, or stirred into smoothies.

**Makes 2 cups**

## INGREDIENTS

1 cup blackberries

1 cup blueberries

½ cup red or black grapes, halved

¼ cup water

1 tbsp lemon juice

1 tsp monk fruit sweetener (optional)

1 tsp fresh ginger, grated

½ tsp ground cinnamon

½ tsp lemon zest

½ tsp vanilla extract

## METHOD

In a saucepan over medium heat, combine all the ingredients and stir well. Bring to a simmer and cook for 10–15 minutes, stirring occasionally, until the berries soften and release their juices.

Mash the mixture slightly with a fork for a textured compote or blend for a smoother consistency. Remove from heat and let cool before serving.

Store in an airtight container in the fridge for up to 5 days.

## *SERVING SUGGESTIONS*

Spoon over coconut yogurt, porridge or pancakes.

Use as a topping for chia pudding or overnight oats.

Blend into smoothies for a resveratrol boost.

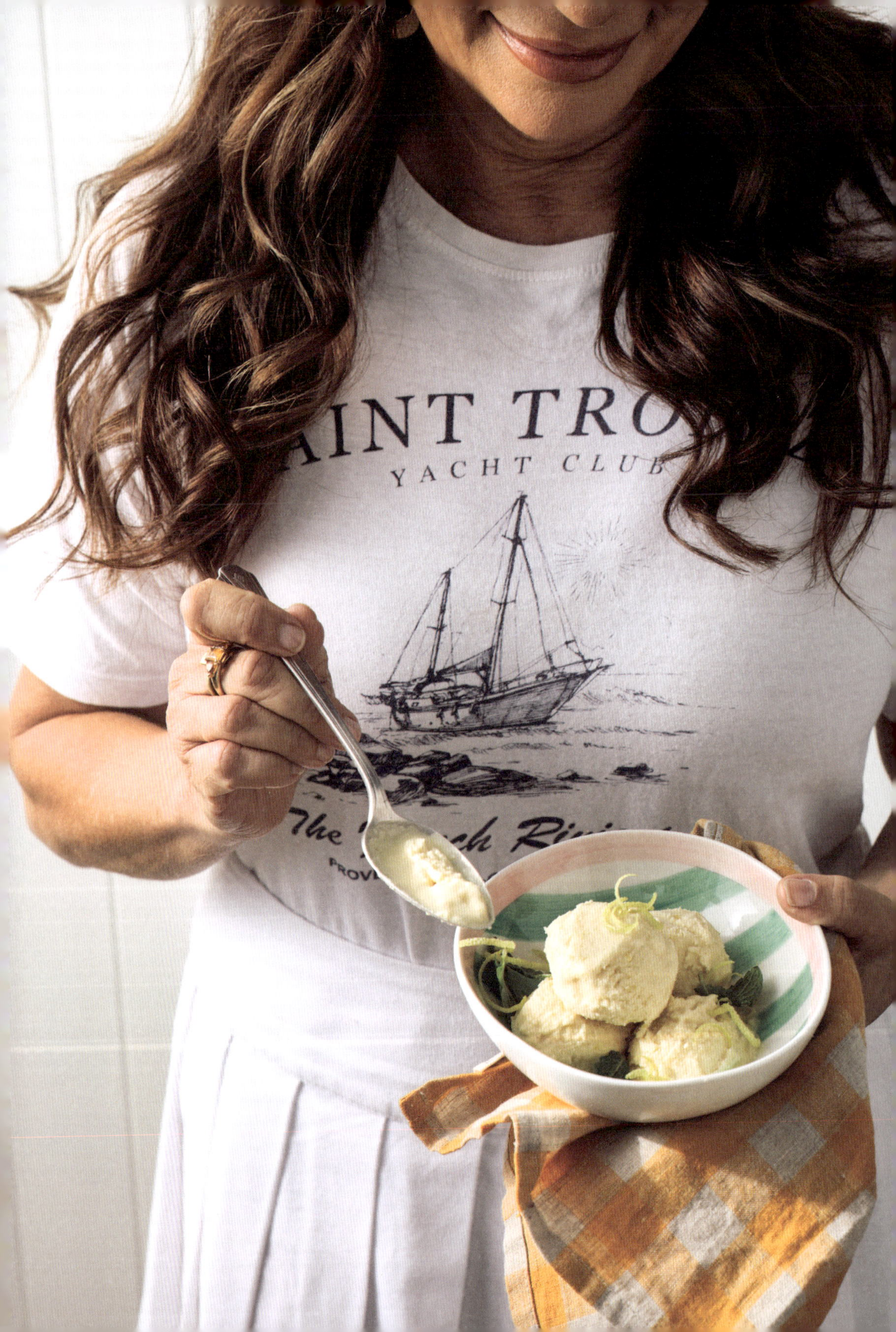
YACHT CLUB

# LEMON & OLIVE OIL ICE CREAM

Enjoy a Mediterranean-inspired frozen treat that's creamy, zesty, and rich in anti-inflammatory fats and gut-friendly protein. Cottage cheese delivers a light, tangy base, while extra virgin olive oil brings silkiness and phytonutrients. A drizzle of olive oil and lemon zest at the end elevates this dessert into something surprisingly elegant.

**Serves 4**

## INGREDIENTS

1½ cups full-fat cottage cheese

3 tbsp pure maple syrup (or to taste)

2 tbsp high-quality extra virgin olive oil (plus extra to drizzle)

1 tbsp freshly squeezed lemon juice

Zest of 1 lemon, plus extra to garnish

1 tsp pure vanilla extract

Flaky sea salt

## METHOD

In a food processor or high-speed blender, combine the cottage cheese, maple syrup, olive oil, lemon juice and zest, vanilla, and sea salt. Blend until completely smooth and creamy.

Pour the mixture into a freezer-safe container. Smooth the top and cover. Freeze for at least 3–4 hours or until firm enough to scoop. (For a creamier texture, stir once or twice during freezing.)

Before serving, let it soften slightly at room temperature for 5–10 minutes.

Scoop into bowls, drizzle lightly with olive oil, and garnish with more lemon zest and a small pinch of flaky sea salt.

# ADAPTOGENIC HERBAL TEA BLEND

This soothing herbal tea blend is infused with adaptogens, which help the body manage stress and inflammation. Ingredients like ashwagandha, tulsi (holy basil) and liquorice root support your adrenal health and immune function, while cinnamon and ginger add warmth and digestive benefits. This blend is perfect for winding down at night or for afternoon stress relief.

***Cooking tip:*** *Liquorice root may not be suitable for people with high blood pressure.*

**Serves 2**

## INGREDIENTS

1 tsp dried ashwagandha
1 tsp dried tulsi (holy basil)
½ tsp dried liquorice root
½ tsp fresh ginger, sliced
½ tsp ground cinnamon
2 cups hot water
1 tsp date syrup (optional)
½ tsp lemon juice

## METHOD

In a teapot or saucepan, combine all the dried herbs and spices. Pour over hot, but not boiling water and let steep for 10–15 minutes.

Strain into two cups and add date syrup (if using) and lemon juice. Enjoy warm for its relaxation and anti-inflammatory benefits.

*OPTIONAL ADDITIONS*

Add a pinch of black pepper to help the adaptogens absorb.

Include dried rose petals for a floral note.

# HEALING HERB & SPICE BLEND

This versatile spice mix is packed with anti-inflammatory ingredients that you can add to soups, stews, roasted vegetables and even salad dressings. Turmeric, cumin and ginger work synergistically to support digestion, reduce inflammation and boost immunity. It's great in a chicken or lentil curry, or tossed with roasted sweet potatoes.

***Cooking tip:*** *Make up large batches of the blend and store in a glass jar to preserve freshness.*

**Makes about ½ cup**

## INGREDIENTS

1 tbsp ground coriander
1 tbsp ground cumin
1 tbsp ground turmeric
1 tsp ground ginger
1 tsp smoked paprika
1 tsp dried rosemary, crushed
1 tsp dried thyme
½ tsp ground cinnamon
½ tsp freshly ground black pepper
½ tsp sea salt

## METHOD

In a small bowl, mix all the ingredients thoroughly. Store in an airtight jar for up to 3 months.

*WAYS TO USE*

Sprinkle over roasted vegetables.

Stir into soups, stews or curries.

Mix with olive oil and lemon juice for a zesty marinade.

Add to scrambled eggs or hummus for extra flavour.

# GLUTEN-FREE OAT & ALMOND-FLOUR BREAD

A wholesome, fibre-rich and gluten-free alternative to traditional loaves. Almond flour and oats meet gut-friendly seeds, adding omega-3s. Perfect for breakfast toast, sandwiches or as a side with soups and salads. Experiment with adding cinnamon or vanilla to bring out the flavour.

***Cooking tip:*** *This loaf is naturally dense; for a lighter texture, try adding ½ teaspoon apple cider vinegar to the batter.*

**Makes 1 loaf**

## INGREDIENTS

3 cups almond flour
1½ cups rolled oats (certified gluten-free)
2 tbsp chia seeds
2 tbsp linseeds (flaxseeds)
3 tsp baking powder (aluminium-free)
¾ tsp sea salt
6 large eggs

## METHOD

Preheat the oven to 175°C (350°F). Grease a standard loaf tin 23 x 13 mm (9 x 5 inches) with cooking spray or melted coconut oil.

In a mixing bowl, combine the almond flour, oats, chia seeds, linseeds, baking powder and salt. Mix well. Add the eggs and stir until a thick, sticky batter forms.

Pour batter into the prepared loaf tin and smooth the top. Bake for 40–50 minutes or until golden brown and a toothpick comes out clean.

Let cool in the tin for 10–15 minutes, then transfer to a wire rack to cool completely. Slice and enjoy with your favourite toppings.

---

*STORAGE*

Store in an airtight container at room temperature for up to 3 days.

Refrigerate for to 1 week for extended freshness.

Slice and freeze with baking (parchment) paper between slices for easy toasting.

# SLOW-COOKED CHICKEN BONE BROTH

Slow-cooked chicken broth is a foundational staple – deeply nourishing, it's full of collagen, gelatine and minerals that support your gut, joint and skin health. Roasting the bones first brings out a rich, savoury depth then the long, low simmer gently extracts vital nutrients without damaging them. Sip it warm with a pinch of sea salt and swirl of olive oil, or use it as a nutrient-dense base for soups, grains and sauces.

**Makes about 2.5–3 litres (2½–3 quarts)**

### INGREDIENTS

1 organic chicken carcass or 2–3 frames, skin and meat remnants intact

2 carrots, chopped

2 celery stalks, chopped

1 leek or onion, quartered

4 cloves garlic, smashed

1 small piece fresh ginger (5 cm/2 inches), sliced

1 small turmeric root (or ½ tsp ground turmeric, optional)

1 tbsp apple cider vinegar

1 tsp whole black peppercorns

1 tsp sea salt

1–2 sprigs fresh rosemary or thyme

Handful of parsley or coriander stalks

2 bay leaves

Filtered water, to cover

### METHOD

Preheat the oven to 200°C (400°F). Spread the chicken bones on a baking tray and roast for 25–30 minutes until deeply golden.

Transfer the bones to a slow cooker. Add all the remaining ingredients. Pour in filtered water until everything is just covered by about 5 cm.

Cook on low for 12–24 hours, leaving the lid slightly ajar. Skim any foam in the first few hours. Leaving the lid ajar helps create a clearer broth, but be aware the liquid will reduce. You can top it up with a little hot water if the level drops below the ingredients.

Let cool slightly, then strain through a fine mesh sieve, discarding the solids. Chill and store. A jelly-like texture once cold means it has a high collagen content. Store in the fridge for 5 days or freeze in portions for up to 3 months.

# SPICED NUT & SEED DUKKAH SPRINKLE

A fragrant, crunchy Egyptian-inspired blend of nuts, seeds and warming spices, dukkah is rich in healthy fats, plant-based protein, fibre and antioxidants. It delivers heart-healthy monounsaturated fats from almonds and walnuts, immune-supporting zinc from pumpkin seeds (pepitas), and anti-inflammatory phytonutrients like cumin and coriander. High in fibre and essential minerals, this dukkah supports digestion, brain health and balanced blood glucose. Use it to add texture, flavour and a nutritional boost to salads, roasted veggies, soups and dips. Store in an airtight jar in the pantry for easy, everyday use.

**Makes about 1 cup**

### INGREDIENTS

½ cup raw almonds
¼ cup raw hazelnuts
3 tbsp pumpkin seeds (pepitas)
3 tbsp sesame seeds (black, white or mixed)
1 tbsp coriander seeds
1 tsp cumin seeds
1 tsp fennel seeds (optional)
½ tsp freshly ground black pepper
½ tsp sea salt
½ tsp smoked paprika or sweet paprika
¼ tsp cayenne pepper (optional)

### METHOD

Preheat the oven to 160°C (320°F). Line a baking tray with baking (parchment) paper.

Spread the almonds and hazelnuts on the lined tray and roast for 10–12 minutes until fragrant and lightly golden. Let cool slightly.

In a dry frying pan (skillet) over medium heat, toast the pumpkin, sesame, coriander, cumin and fennel seeds until aromatic (2–3 minutes), stirring frequently. Remove from heat and cool.

In a food processor or using a mortar and pestle, pulse the nuts and seeds in batches until coarsely chopped. Aim for a mix of fine and chunky textures, not a powder.

Transfer to a bowl then mix in the pepper, salt, paprika and cayenne (if using). Adjust seasoning to taste. Store in an airtight jar at room temperature for up to 3 weeks.

# ANTI-INFLAMMATORY RECIPES

## BREAKFASTS 142



## LUNCHES 161

## DINNERS 194



## DESSERTS, SNACKS AND SAVOURIES 227

# APPENDIX 1. COMPREHENSIVE MAP SHOPPING LIST

## FRUITS

Apples
Apricots
Avocados
Bananas (slightly green for resistant starch)
Blackberries
Blueberries frozen berries
Cherries (especially tart varieties)
Clementines
Dates and medjool dates
Dried apricots (without sulfur)
Dried blueberries (unsweetened)
Figs (fresh and dried)
Frozen berries
Goji berries
Grapes (red or black)
Lemons and preserved lemons
Limes
Melons (watermelon, rockmelon/cantaloupe, honeydew melon)
Nectarines
Papaya
Passionfruit
Pineapple
Pears
Pomegranate (whole and seeds)
Raspberries
Tomatoes (can be inflammatory so use with caution)

## VEGETABLES

Artichokes
Asparagus
Beetroot (beets)
Broccoli and broccoli sprouts
Brussels sprouts
Cabbage
Carrots
Cauliflower (including cauliflower rice)
Celery
Chicory root
Cucumber
Endive
Fennel bulb
Garlic
Green beans
Jerusalem artichokes
Kale
Leeks
Lemongrass
Mixed leaves
Mushrooms (plus other medicinal varieties)
Okra
Onions (red, yellow, small, spring onions, shallots)
Pumpkin and winter squashes
Purple cabbage
Radicchio
Radishes
Rocket (arugula)
Silverbeet (Swiss chard)
Spinach
Sweet potatoes
Turnips
Watercress
Zucchini (courgette)

## FRESH HERBS & AROMATICS

Basil and holy basil
Bay leaves
Chives
Coriander (cilantro)
Fresh ginger
Fresh turmeric
Green chillies
Mint
Parsley
Rosemary
Sage
Thyme

## SPICES & DRIED HERBS

Ashwagandha root
Black pepper
Cacao powder
Cardamom
Cayenne pepper
Chilli
Cinnamon
Cloves
Coriander seeds
Cumin
Dukkah seasoning
Fenugreek
Garlic powder
Ginger
Liquorice root
Mixed and dried herbs
Marjoram

Nutmeg
Onion powder
Oregano
Paprika (smoked)
Saffron
Sea salt
Sumac
Sweet paprika
Thyme
Turmeric
Za'atar spice blend

## NUTS & SEEDS

Almonds (raw and blanched)
Brazil nuts
Chia seeds
Hemp seeds
Linseeds (flaxseeds), ground
Macadamias
Nut butters (with nuts listed)
Pecans
Pumpkin seeds (pepitas)
Pine nuts
Pistachios
Sesame seeds (black and white)
Tiger nuts
Walnuts

## PROTEIN & DAIRY

Anchovies
Bone broth (chicken or beef, ideally homemade)
Beef (grass-fed, occasionally, no more than once per fortnight)
Chicken (free-range, organic, cubed and bone-in options)
Cottage cheese
Eggs (pasture-raised when possible)
Feta
Goat's and sheep's cheese (soft and hard varieties)
Goat's milk
Labneh
Lamb shoulder (grass-fed, occasionally, no more than once per week)
Mackerel fillets
Milk (A2 in moderation)
Mozzarella (fresh in moderation)
Parmesan
Ricotta (in moderation)
Salmon (wild)
Sardines
Smoked trout
Supercharged Food Vanilla Protein Powder
Tzatziki
Tempeh and tofu (organic, non-GMO)
Venison (occasionally)
White fish (haddock, sea bass, plaice)
Yogurt (Greek, sheep's, plain)

## GRAINS & LEGUMES

Adzuki beans
Ancient grains
Amaranth
Barley
Black beans
Buckwheat
Brown rice
Chickpeas (garbanzo beans), dried and canned
Gluten-free oats
Farro
Kidney beans
Lentils (red, green, black)
Millet
Mung beans
Oats (oatmeal)
Quinoa
Sorghum
Split peas
Teff
Tempeh
Tofu
Wild rice

## SUPERFOODS & ADDITIONS

Acerola cherry
Cacao nibs
Camu camu
Coconut flakes
Crispy shallots
Dark chocolate (85% cacao or higher)
Love Your Gut Fulvic Humic Concentrate
Love Your Gut Protein and Fibre
Love Your Gut Super Potent Curcumin
Love Your Gut Synbiotic powder or capsules
Microgreens or sprouts
Nutritional yeast flakes
Popcorn (natural)
Protein powder (unsweetened, plant-based or collagen)
Puffed cereal

## PANTRY STAPLES & CONDIMENTS

Almond butter (unsweetened)
Almond flour/meal
Apple cider vinegar (raw, unfiltered)
Baking powder (aluminium-free)
Brown rice flour
Capers
Chickpea (garbanzo bean) flour
Coconut aminos or tamari
Coconut milk (full-fat, BPA-free cans)
Coconut oil (virgin, unrefined)
Coconut yogurt (unsweetened)
Dijon mustard
Dried raspberries
Maple syrup (small amounts)
Monk fruit extract and sweetener
Plant-based milks (nut and oat milks)
Sea salt
Sorghum flour
Tahini (unsweetened)
Tortilla chips (natural)
Vanilla extract (pure)
Yacon syrup

## OILS & VINEGARS

Apple cider vinegar
Avocado oil
Coconut oil
Extra virgin olive oil (cold-pressed, high-quality)
Linseed (flaxseed) oil (refrigerated)
Hemp oil
MCT oil
Perilla oil

## FERMENTED FOODS

Capers
Cultured cheese
Greek yogurt
Kefir
Olives and fermented olives
Pickled vegetables
Sauerkraut
Tempeh

## BEVERAGES

Dandelion tea
Green tea
Herbal teas (tulsi, peppermint, chamomile, ginger)
Tart cherry juice (unsweetened)
Red wine (occasionally)

# APPENDIX 2. A NOTE ON DAIRY IN ANTI-INFLAMMATORY EATING

Dairy deserves special consideration in an anti-inflammatory diet. While some modern approaches eliminate dairy entirely, traditional Mediterranean diets have always included specific dairy foods in moderate amounts. Fermented options like yogurt and certain cheeses (especially goat's and sheep's cheeses), tend to be better tolerated and potentially less inflammatory than conventional cow's dairy. These products contain A2 casein protein rather than the A1 casein found in most cow's milk, which may improve their digestibility and reduce inflammatory potential.

Mozzarella and ricotta both have a place on the anti-inflammatory Mediterranean table because they're fresh, minimally processed cheeses that sidestep many of the inflammatory triggers found in their heavily processed, aged counterparts. Unlike mature cheeses that can spike histamine levels and inflammatory responses, these gentle varieties are naturally lower in histamines and easier on sensitive systems. Ricotta brings an additional bonus with its whey protein content, which actually possesses anti-inflammatory properties along with delivering high-quality protein. When sourced from grass-fed animals, these cheeses also provide beneficial omega-3 fatty acids that support your body's natural anti-inflammatory processes.

Hard cheeses such as parmesan can contain very little lactose, making them potentially more easily digestible and less likely to cause inflammation-associated digestive issues. Parmigiano Reggiano, a type of parmesan, contains peptides with immune-regulating properties regulatory activities, which can help regulate the immune system. Parmesan contains butyrate, a short-chain fatty acid that can induce modulatory activities on the immune system).

The Mediterranean approach isn't about eliminating entire food groups but choosing the highest quality versions and enjoying them as part of a predominantly plant-based diet. These cheeses work brilliantly in dishes like ricotta-stuffed courgette flowers, fresh mozzarella with tomatoes and basil, or ricotta mixed with herbs as a spread. Quality matters tremendously – opt for organic, grass-fed sources whenever possible because these have higher omega-3 content. Use dairy thoughtfully as flavour enhancers or accompaniments rather than dietary staples, and pay attention to your body's individual response because tolerance varies significantly from person to person. For many, high-quality fermented dairy in modest amounts can be a delightful and nutritious component of an anti-inflammatory Mediterranean diet.

## APPENDIX 3. YOUR NUTRIENT GUIDEBOOK TO CONQUER INFLAMMATION

The following table lists the key anti-inflammatory compounds, nutrients and supplements discussed in this chapter. I've compiled this alphabetical guide to help you quickly identify what each substance does, where it works in the body, why it's beneficial for managing inflammation and how to incorporate it into your health regimen.

Remember, while this table offers valuable guidance, you should work with a healthcare practitioner or clinical nutritionist to create a personalised protocol based on your unique biochemistry and health goals.

## COMMON NUTRIENTS AND SUPPLEMENTS

| NUTRIENT/ SUPPLEMENT | WHERE IT ACTS | WHY IT'S GOOD FOR YOU | SOURCE |
|---|---|---|---|
| **Allicin** | Immune system | Enhances immune modulation and reduces oxidative stress | Raw garlic, fermented garlic preparations |
| **Anthocyanins** | Vascular system, cellular protection | Lower oxidative stress, improve vascular function | Blueberries, blackberries, purple/red fruits |
| **Apple cider vinegar** | Digestive system, metabolic pathways | Supports digestion, improves insulin sensitivity | Fermented apple products, supplemental capsules |
| **Ashwagandha** | Hypothalamic–pituitary–adrenal axis | Modulates stress response and mitigates stress-related gut dysfunction | Herbal supplement, adaptogenic formulas |
| **Bromelain** | Systemic circulation, inflammatory sites | Proteolytic enzyme that breaks down inflammatory proteins | Pineapple (especially stems), supplemental form |
| **Butyrate** | Colon, gut barrier | Strengthens gut barrier, reduces intestinal inflammation, regulates T-regulatory cells | Produced by gut bacteria from fermentable fibre; resistant starch in cooked then cooled potatoes, green bananas |
| **Carnitine** | Mitochondria | Facilitates fatty acid transport for energy production | Red meat, supplemental form |
| **Carnosic acid** | Cellular antioxidant systems | Activates nuclear factor erythroid 2-related factor 2 (Nrf2) pathway, enhances cellular defences | Rosemary, sage |
| **Carotenoids** | Cell membranes, tissue protection | Act as potent antioxidants | Sweet potatoes, carrots, capsicums (bell peppers), other brightly coloured fruits and vegetables |
| **Collagen** | Connective tissue, gut lining | Supports joint health, gut integrity, skin elasticity | Bone broth, supplemental forms |
| **Coenzyme $Q_{10}$ ($CoQ_{10}$)** | Mitochondrial electron transport chain | Supports cellular energy production, antioxidant | Organ meats, oily fish, supplemental form |
| **Creatine** | Muscle energy systems | Supports cellular energy production | Animal products, supplemental form |

## COMMON NUTRIENTS AND SUPPLEMENTS

| NUTRIENT/ SUPPLEMENT | WHERE IT ACTS | WHY IT'S GOOD FOR YOU | SOURCE |
|---|---|---|---|
| **Curcumin** | Active compound in turmeric | Blocks nuclear factor kappa B (NF-κB), reduces cyclooxygenase-2 (COX-2) activity, inhibits pro-inflammatory cytokines like tumour necrosis factor (TNF) | Love Your Gut Super Potent Curcumin with Black Pepper |
| **Diatomaceous earth** | Digestive tract | Helps cleanse digestive system, supports microbiome balance | Love Your Gut Powder |
| **Flavonoids** | Inflammatory cascade | Reduce inflammatory mediators like TNF and interleukin-6 | Citrus fruits, onions, tea |
| **Fulvic humic concentrate** | Cellular mineral transport | Aids mineral absorption, detoxification, cellular energy | Love Your Gut Fulvic Humic Concentrate |
| **Ginger compounds (gingerols/shogaols)** | Anti-inflammatory pathways | Inhibits inflammatory enzymes similar to pharmaceutical anti-inflammatories | Fresh ginger root, ginger tea |
| **Glycine** | Connective tissue, nervous system | Helps repair gut lining integrity | Collagen, bone broth |
| **Golden gut blend** | Digestive system, gut health | Supports gut cleansing, reduces inflammation, enhances nutrient absorption | Turmeric, spices, diatomaceous earth; used in lattes, smoothies, porridge, etc. |
| **L-glutamine** | Gut lining, muscle tissue | Supports gut barrier repair and reduces permeability | Bone broth, meat |
| **Magnesium** | Nervous system, muscle function | Relaxes nervous system and reduces gut spasms | Dark leafy greens, nuts, seeds, supplemental forms |
| **Maresins** | Sites of inflammation | Specialised pro-resolving mediator that actively resolves inflammation | Derived from DHA (an omega-3 fatty acid), supplemental form |
| **N-acetylcysteine (NAC)** | Cellular detoxification | Supports glutathione production, reduces oxidative stress | Supplemental form |
| **Nattokinase** | Circulatory system | Fibrinolytic enzyme that breaks down inflammatory proteins and improves circulation | Natto (fermented soybeans), supplemental form |

## COMMON NUTRIENTS AND SUPPLEMENTS

| NUTRIENT/ SUPPLEMENT | WHERE IT ACTS | WHY IT'S GOOD FOR YOU | SOURCE |
|---|---|---|---|
| **Omega-3 fatty acids: eicosapentaenoic acid (EPA) and docosahexaenoic acid (DHA)** | Cell membranes, neural tissue | Reduces inflammation by suppressing pro-inflammatory prostaglandins and leukotrienes | Wild-caught salmon, mackerel, linseeds (flaxseeds), walnuts, algae-based supplements |
| **Palmitoylethanolamide (PEA)** | Nervous system, mast cells | Reduces neuroinflammation and mast cell activation | Supplemental form |
| **Papain** | Systemic circulation, joints | Proteolytic enzyme that reduces inflammatory proteins | Papaya, supplemental form |
| **Polyphenols** | Cellular signalling pathways | Regulate inflammatory gene expression | Berries, green tea, dark chocolate, extra virgin olive oil |
| **Pyrroloquinoline quinone (PQQ)** | Mitochondria | Supports mitochondrial biogenesis and function | Fermented foods, supplemental form |
| **Prebiotics** | Gut microbiome | Feed beneficial bacteria that produce anti-inflammatory compounds | Onions, garlic, bananas, Jerusalem artichokes |
| **Probiotics (specific strains)** | Gut microbiome | Modulate immune function, produce anti-inflammatory compounds | Fermented foods, targeted probiotic supplements |
| **Protectins** | Neural tissue, sites of inflammation | Specialised pro-resolving mediator that protects tissue during inflammation | Derived from DHA (an omega-3 fatty acid); supplemental form |
| **Pterostilbene** | Cellular antioxidant systems | Activates Nrf2 pathway, enhances cellular defences | Blueberries, supplemental form |
| **Quercetin** | Cell membranes, inflammatory cascades | Natural antihistamine, stabilises mast cells | Onions, apples, capers, supplemental form |
| **Resolvins** | Sites of inflammation | Specialised pro-resolving mediator that actively resolves inflammation | Derived from EPA and DHA (omega-3 fatty acids), supplemental form |
| **Resveratrol** | Cellular signalling pathways | Activates sirtuin pathways, reduces oxidative damage | Red grapes, berries, dark chocolate, red wine |
| **Rhodiola** | Hypothalamic–pituitary–adrenal axis axis | Modulates stress response and supports cellular energy | Herbal supplement, adaptogenic formulas |

## COMMON NUTRIENTS AND SUPPLEMENTS

| NUTRIENT/ SUPPLEMENT | WHERE IT ACTS | WHY IT'S GOOD FOR YOU | SOURCE |
|---|---|---|---|
| **Serrapeptase** | Systemic circulation, inflammatory sites | Proteolytic enzyme that reduces inflammation and pain | Supplemental form |
| **Short-chain fatty acids** | Colon, immune system | Support gut barrier, regulate immune function | Produced by gut bacteria from fermentable fibre |
| **Sulforaphane** | Cellular detoxification pathways | Enhances detoxification and cellular defence mechanisms against oxidative stress | Broccoli sprouts, cruciferous vegetables |
| **Synbiotic formula** | Gut microbiome | Beneficial combination of probiotics, prebiotics, digestive enzymes and dietary fibre; optimises gut health and immune function | Love Your Gut Synbiotic |
| **Triterpenoids** | Cellular antioxidant systems | Activate Nrf2 pathway, potent anti-inflammatory | Olives, olive oil, many medicinal herbs |
| **Vitamin D** | Immune cells, gut barrier | Regulates immune function, supports gut barrier | Sunlight exposure, fatty fish, supplemental form |
| **Zinc** | Immune cells, enzyme systems | Supports immune function, wound healing | Oysters, red meat, pumpkin seeds (pepitas) |

Peptides are short chains of amino acids that act as powerful signalling molecules in the body, influencing everything from muscle repair and skin health to gut integrity and inflammation control. They're found naturally in foods like collagen, dairy, fish and plants, and are also available in targeted therapeutic forms such as BPC-157. The following table highlights some of the most common peptides used to support your overall health and wellbeing.

## COMMON BIOACTIVE AND THERAPEUTIC PEPTIDES

| PEPTIDES | WHERE IT ACTS | WHY IT'S GOOD FOR YOU | SOURCE |
|---|---|---|---|
| **BPC-157** | Systemically, targeting gut, muscle and tendon tissues. | Promotes rapid tissue healing and reduces systemic inflammation | Not found in food; supplemental form |
| **Collagen peptides** | Joints, gut lining, skin and connective tissues | Strengthens the gut barrier and supports joint health to reduce sources of inflammation | Bone broth, skin-on chicken, fish skin, gelatine, tough cuts of meat |
| **Dairy peptides** | Systemically throughout the body via the bloodstream | Has antioxidant and anti-inflammatory effects | Greek yogurt, kefir, cottage cheese, milk |
| **Fish peptides** | Systemically throughout the body via the bloodstream. | Offers potent antioxidant and anti-inflammatory benefits, particularly for skin and joints | Salmon, mackerel, sardines (especially with skin), fish-head broth |
| **Plant-based peptides** | Systemically throughout the body via the bloodstream | Helps to reduce inflammation and provides antioxidant support | Lentils, chickpeas, peas, soy (tofu, edamame), hemp seeds |
| **Thymosin beta-4 (TB-500)** | Systemically; acts on virtually all cells in the body. | Supports cell regeneration, wound repair and modulates the inflammatory response | Not found in food; supplemental form |

# ANNOTATED BIBLIOGRAPHY

## Chapter 3: What causes chronic inflammation

**Processed foods and C-reactive protein (CRP):** Diets high in processed foods can increase inflammatory markers.

Lane, M. M., Lotfaliany, M., Forbes, M., Loughman, A., Rocks, T., O'Neil, A., Machado, P., Jacka, F. N., Hodge, A., & Marx, W. (2022). Higher ultra-processed food consumption is associated with greater high-sensitivity C-reactive protein concentration in adults: Cross-sectional results from the Melbourne Collaborative Cohort Study. *Nutrients, 14*(16), 3309. https://pubmed.ncbi.nlm.nih.gov/36014818/

## Chapter 4: How chronic inflammation disrupts health from head to toe

**C-reactive protein (CRP) and heart attack risk:** High CRP levels are a risk factor for heart attacks, even with normal cholesterol.

Amezcua-Castillo, E., González-Pacheco, H., Sáenz-San Martín, A., Méndez-Ocampo, P., Gutierrez-Moctezuma, I., Massó, F., Sierra-Lara, D., Springall, R., Rodríguez, E., Arias-Mendoza, A., & Amezcua-Guerra, L. M. (2023). C-reactive protein: The quintessential marker of systemic inflammation in coronary artery disease – advancing toward precision medicine. *Biomedicines, 11*(9), 2444. https://pmc.ncbi.nlm.nih.gov/articles/PMC10525787/

**Rudolf Virchow's historical observation:** The 19th-century observation of inflammatory cells in atherosclerotic plaques.

Libby, P. (2012). Inflammation in atherosclerosis. Arteriosclerosis, *Thrombosis, and Vascular Biology,* 32(9), 2045–2051. https://www.ahajournals.org/doi/10.1161/atvbaha.108.179705

**Inflammation as a driver of atherosclerosis:** Inflammation is a central orchestrator of all stages of atherosclerosis.

Libby, P. (2002). Inflammation in atherosclerosis. Nature, *420*(6917), 868–874. https://pubmed.ncbi.nlm.nih.gov/12490960/

**Trimethylamine N-oxide (TMAO) and cardiovascular disease:** The gut-derived metabolite TMAO is associated with an increased risk of atherosclerotic cardiovascular disease.

Tang, W. H., Wang, Z., Levison, B. S., Koeth, R. A., Britt, E. B., Fu, X., Wu, Y., & Hazen, S. L. (2013). Intestinal microbial metabolism of phosphatidylcholine and cardiovascular risk. *The New England Journal of Medicine, 368, 1575–1584.* https://www.nejm.org/doi/full/10.1056/nejmoa1109400

**CANTOS Trial (2017):** A clinical trial demonstrating that targeting inflammation with canakinumab reduces the risk of cardiovascular events.

Baylis, R. A., Gomez, D., Mallat, Z., Pasterkamp, G., & Owens, G. K. (2017). The CANTOS Trial: One important step for clinical cardiology but a giant leap for vascular biology. Arteriosclerosis, *Thrombosis, and Vascular Biology,* 37(11), e174–e177. https://pmc.ncbi.nlm.nih.gov/articles/PMC5685554/

**Inflammation and mood disorders:** Chronic inflammation is involved in mood disorders like depression and anxiety.

Felger, J. C. (2018). Imaging the role of inflammation in mood and anxiety-related disorders. *Current Neuropharmacology, 16*(5), 533–558. https://pmc.ncbi.nlm.nih.gov/articles/PMC5997866

**Gut microbiome and neurotransmitter production:** Gut bacteria are involved in the production of key neurotransmitters.

Appleton, J. (2018). The gut-brain axis: Influence of microbiota on mood and mental health. I*ntegrative Medicine (Encinitas, Calif.), 17*(4), 28–32. https://pmc.ncbi.nlm.nih.gov/articles/PMC6469458/

**Diet, neuroinflammation and depression:** High-sugar diets are linked to depression and anti-inflammatory diets protect against mood disorders.

Jacques, A., Chaaya, N., Beecher, K., Ali, S. A., Belmer, A., & Bartlett, S. (2019). The impact of sugar consumption on stress driven, emotional and addictive behaviors. *Neuroscience & Biobehavioral Reviews,* 103, 178–199. https://www.sciencedirect.com/science/article/pii/S0149763418308613

**Inflammation and Alzheimer's disease: A** link between higher levels of systemic inflammation and an increased risk of developing Alzheimer's disease.

Akiyama, H., Barger, S., Barnum, S., Bradt, B., Bauer, J., Cole, G. M., Cooper, N. R., Eikelenboom, P., Emmerling, M., Fiebich, B. L., Finch, C. E., Frautschy, S., Griffin, W. S., Hampel, H., Hull, M., Landreth, G., Lue, L., Mrak, R., Mackenzie, I. R., McGeer, P. L., ... Wyss-Coray, T. (2000). Inflammation and Alzheimer's disease. *Neurobiology of Aging, 21*(3), 383–421. https://pmc.ncbi.nlm.nih.gov/articles/PMC3887148/

**Brain fog, inflammation and mitochondrial dysfunction:** Cognitive impairment systemic inflammation and mitochondrial dysfunction.

Wang, Q., Lu, M., Zhu, X., Gu, X., Zhang, T., Xia, C., Yang, L., Xu, Y., & Zhou, M. (2022). Brain mitochondrial dysfunction: A possible mechanism links early life anxiety to Alzheimer's disease in later life. *Aging and Disease, 13*(4), 1127–1145. https://pmc.ncbi.nlm.nih.gov/articles/PMC9286915

**Inflammation and polycystic ovary syndrome (PCOS):** Linking chronic inflammation to PCOS and its associated insulin resistance.

González, F. (2012). Inflammation in polycystic ovary syndrome: Underpinning of insulin resistance and ovarian dysfunction. *Steroids, 77*(4), 300–305. https://pmc.ncbi.nlm.nih.gov/articles/PMC3309040

***Prevotella copri* in rheumatoid arthritis:** A distinct gut microbiome profile in individuals with rheumatoid arthritis, often characterised by an overabundance of *Prevotella copri.*

Scher, J. U., Sczesnak, A., Longman, R. S., Segata, N., Ubeda, C., Bielski, C., Rostron, T., Cerundolo, V., Pamer, E. G., Abramson, S. B., Huttenhower, C., Littman, D. R. (2013). Expansion of intestinal *Prevotella copri* correlates with enhanced susceptibility to arthritis. *eLife, 2,* e01202. https://elifesciences.org/articles/01202

**Gut bacterial DNA in synovial fluid:** The DNA of gut bacteria within the joint fluid of patients with rheumatoid arthritis.

Scher, J. U., Sczesnak, A., Longman, R. S., Segata, N., Ubeda, C., Bielski, C., Rostron, T., Cerundolo, V., Pamer, E. G., Abramson, S. B., Huttenhower, C., Littman, D. R. (2013). Expansion of intestinal *Prevotella copri* correlates with enhanced susceptibility to arthritis. *eLife, 2,* e01202. https://elifesciences.org/articles/01202

**Systemic lupus erythematosus (SLE) progression patterns:** Identifying four distinct patterns of disease progression in lupus.

Parodis, I., Lindblom, J., Tsoi, A., Palazzo, L., Blomkvist Sporre, K., Enman, Y., Nikolopoulos, D., Beretta, L. (2025). Trajectories of disease evolution upon treatment initiation in systemic lupus erythematosus: Results from four clinical trials of belimumab. *Rheumatology, 64*(5), 2697–2705. https://academic.oup.com/rheumatology/article/64/5/2697/7824072#google_vignette

**Gut–brain axis in multiple sclerosis (MS):** The role of the gut microbiome and its connection to the brain in exacerbating neuroinflammation in MS.

Takewaki, D., & Yamamura, T. (2021). Gut microbiome research in multiple sclerosis. *Neuroscience Research, 168*, 28–31. https://www.sciencedirect.com/science/article/abs/pii/S0168010221000973

## Chapter 5: Your gut is command central

**Artificial sweeteners and gut microbiome:** Artificial sweeteners can reduce populations of beneficial bacteria.

Ruiz-Ojeda, F. J., Plaza-Díaz, J., Sáez-Lara, M. J., & Gil, A. (2019). Effects of sweeteners on the gut microbiota: A review of experimental studies and clinical trials. *Advances in Nutrition (Bethesda, Md.), 10(suppl_1), S31–S48.* https://pmc.ncbi.nlm.nih.gov/articles/PMC6363527/

**Prebiotic fibres and beneficial bacteria:** Prebiotic fibres selectively nourish beneficial gut bacteria such as *Bifidobacteria and Akkermansia.*

Davani-Davari, D., Negahdaripour, M., Karimzadeh, I., Seifan, M., Mohkam, M., Masoumi, S. J., Berenjian, A., & Ghasemi, Y. (2019). Prebiotics: Definition, types, sources, mechanisms, and clinical applications. *Foods (Basel, Switzerland), 8*(3), 92. https://pmc.ncbi.nlm.nih.gov/articles/PMC6463098/

## Chapter 6: Your mind–body connection: Healing trauma and stress

**Adverse childhood experiences (ACEs) and irritable bowel syndrome (IBS):** Individuals with a history of ACEs are twice as likely to develop IBS.

Berens, S., Banzhaf, P., Baumeister, D., & Gauss, A. (2019). Relationship between adverse childhood experiences and illness anxiety in irritable bowel syndrome – The impact of gender. *Journal of Psychosomatic Research, 128*(34), 109846. https://www.researchgate.net/publication/336674448

**Chronic stress and gut microbiome:** Chronic stress can reduce beneficial bacteria populations.

Madison, A., & Kiecolt-Glaser, J. K. (2019). Stress, depression, diet, and the gut microbiota: Human-bacteria interactions at the core of psychoneuroimmunology and nutrition. *Current Opinion in Behavioral Sciences, 28*, 105–110. https://pmc.ncbi.nlm.nih.gov/articles/PMC7213601

**Self-compassion meditation and inflammation:** Practising self-compassion can lead to a measurable reduction in inflammatory markers.

Pace, T. W.W., Negi, L. T., Adame, D. D., Cole, S. P., Sivilli, T. I., Brown, T. D., Issa, M. J., Raison, C. L. (2009). Effect of compassion meditation on neuroendocrine, innate immune and behavioral responses to psychosocial stress. *Psychoneuroendocrinology, 34*(1), 87–98. https://www.sciencedirect.com/science/article/abs/pii/S0306453008002199

**Childhood trauma and long-term inflammation:** Adults with a history of childhood trauma have persistently higher levels of inflammatory markers.

Baumeister, D., Akhtar, R., Ciufolini, S., Pariante, C. M., & Mondelli, V. (2016). Childhood trauma and adulthood inflammation: A meta-analysis of peripheral C-reactive protein, interleukin-6 and tumour necrosis factor-α. *Molecular Psychiatry, 21*(5), 642–649. https://pubmed.ncbi.nlm.nih.gov/26033244/

**Polyvagal theory (Dr Stephen Porges):** The theory providing a framework for understanding the body's autonomic nervous system.

Porges, S. W. (2017). *The pocket guide to the polyvagal theory: The transformative power of feeling safe.* W. W. Norton & Company.

**Mindfulness and inflammatory markers:** Individuals who practice mindfulness regularly have lower levels of inflammatory markers.

Pascoe, M. C., de Manincor, M., Tseberja, J., Hallgren, M., Baldwin, P. A., Parker, A. G. (2021). Psychobiological mechanisms underlying the mood benefits of meditation: A narrative review. *Comprehensive Psychoneuroendocrinology, 6,* 100037. https://www.sciencedirect.com/science/article/pii/S2666497621000114

**Brain imaging studies on mindfulness:** Using neuroimaging to show that mindfulness practices lead to structural and functional brain changes.

Fox, K. C. R., Dixon, M. L., Nijeboer, S., Girn, M., Floman, J. L., Lifshitz, M., Ellamil, M., Sedlmeier, P., Christoff, K. (2016). Functional neuroanatomy of meditation: A review and meta-analysis of 78 functional neuroimaging investigations. *Quantitative Biology: Neurons and Cognition,* Cornell University. https://arxiv.org/abs/1603.06342

**Biophilia hypothesis (E. O. Wilson):** Humans have an innate affinity for nature.

Bratman, G. N., Anderson, C. B., Berman, M. G., Cochran, B., de Vries, S., Flanders, J., Folke, C., Frumkin, H., Gross, J. J., Hartig, T., Kahn, P. H., Jr., Kuo, M., Lawler, J. J., Levin, P. S., Lindahl, T., Meyer-Lindenberg, A., Mitchell, R., Ouyang, Z., Roe, J., Scarlett, L., Smith, J. R., van den Bosch, M., Wheeler, B. W., White, M. P., Zheng, H., & Daily, G. C. (2019). Nature and mental health: An ecosystem service perspective. *Science Advances, 5*(7), eaax0903. https://doi.org/10.1126/sciadv.aax0903

## Chapter 10: Targeted nutrition and supplementation to reduce inflammation

**Curcumin versus NSAIDs:** Curcumin can be as effective as NSAIDs for managing inflammatory conditions.

Mohseni, S., Tavakoli, A., Ghazipoor, H., Pouralimohamadi, N., Zare, R., Rampp, T., Shayesteh, M., & Pasalar, M. (2025). Curcumin for the clinical treatment of inflammatory bowel diseases: A systematic review and meta-analysis of placebo-controlled randomized clinical trials. *Frontiers in Nutrition, 12,* 1494351. https://www.frontiersin.org/journals/nutrition/articles/10.3389/fnut.2025.1494351

**Inflammatory bowel disease (IBD) and gut bacteria strains:** Isolated specific gut bacteria strains with the potential to be used in new IBD treatments.

Selvamani, S., Mehta, V., El Enshasy, H. A., Thevarajoo, S., El Adawi, H., Zeini, I., Pham, K., Varzakas, T., & Abomoelak, B. (2022). Efficacy of probiotics-based interventions as therapy for inflammatory bowel disease: A recent update. *Saudi Journal of Biological Sciences, 29*(5), 3546–3567. https://www.sciencedirect.com/science/article/pii/S1319562X22001206

**Psychobiotics and the vagus nerve: Specific probiotic strains** (*Lactobacillus plantarum PS128 and Bifidobacterium longum 1714)* can modulate the vagus nerve.

Cheng, L.-H., Liu, Y.-W., Wu, C.-C., Wang, S., & Tsai, Y.-C. (2019). Psychobiotics in mental health, neurodegenerative and neurodevelopmental disorders. *Journal of Food and Drug Analysis, 27*(3), 632–648. https://www.sciencedirect.com/science/article/pii/S1021949819300158

**Butyrate and gut health:** Multiple anti-inflammatory functions of the short-chain fatty acid butyrate.

Hodgkinson, K., El Abbar, F., Dobranowski, P., Manoogian, J., Butcher, J., Figeys, D., Mack, D., & Stintzi, A. (2023). Butyrate's role in human health and the current progress towards its clinical application to treat gastrointestinal disease. *Clinical Nutrition,* 42(2), 61–75. https://www.sciencedirect.com/science/article/pii/S0261561422003843

## Chapter 11: Navigating the Mediterranean path

**Seven Countries Study (Dr Ancel Keys):** This landmark epidemiological study linked the traditional Mediterranean diet to lower rates of heart disease.

Menotti, A., & Puddu, P. E. (2025). Ancel Keys, the Mediterranean diet, and the Seven Countries Study: A review. *Journal of Cardiovascular Development and Disease,* 12(4), 141. https://pmc.ncbi.nlm.nih.gov/articles/PMC12027923/

**Mediterranean diet and inflammation markers:** A Mediterranean diet supplemented with extra nuts or olive oil lowered markers of inflammation.

Estruch, R., Ros, E., Salas-Salvadó, J., Covas, M.-I., Corella, D., Arós, F., Gómez-Gracia, E., Ruiz-Gutiérrez, V., Fiol, M., Lapetra, J., Lamuela-Raventos, R. M., Serra-Majem, L., Pintó, X., Basora, J., Muñoz, M. A., Sorlí, J. V., Martínez, J. A., Fitó, M., Gea, A., ... Martínez-González, M. A., for the PREDIMED Study Investigators. (2018). Primary prevention of cardiovascular disease with a Mediterranean diet supplemented with extra-virgin olive oil or nuts. *The New England Journal of Medicine,* 378(25), e34. https://www.nejm.org/doi/full/10.1056/NEJMoa1800389

**Chronic disease prevention through diet:** Nutrition and healthy eating habits can reduce the risk or slow the progression of long-term illnesses.

Neuhouser, M. L. (2019). The importance of healthy dietary patterns in chronic disease prevention. *Nutrition Research (New York, N.Y.),* 70, 3–6. https://pubmed.ncbi.nlm.nih.gov/30077352

# ACKNOWLEDGEMENTS

Thank you, Tamsin, my constant sidekick and inspiration. To my friends and family: your love and support ground me every day. At Rockpool Publishing, I'd like to thank Lisa and Paul for championing the concept, and to Raquel, Christine, Sara and Katie for managing every moving piece with such grace and expertise. Jessica Cox, you're a wonderful editor. A special acknowledgement goes to Rob Palmer, Vanessa Austin, Miche Bloch and Emma Norton who made the food look and taste so good. Finally, thanks to Louise Antonjuk for making me look less like I'd been up all night researching glycaemic indices!